THIS JOURNAL
BELONGS TO:

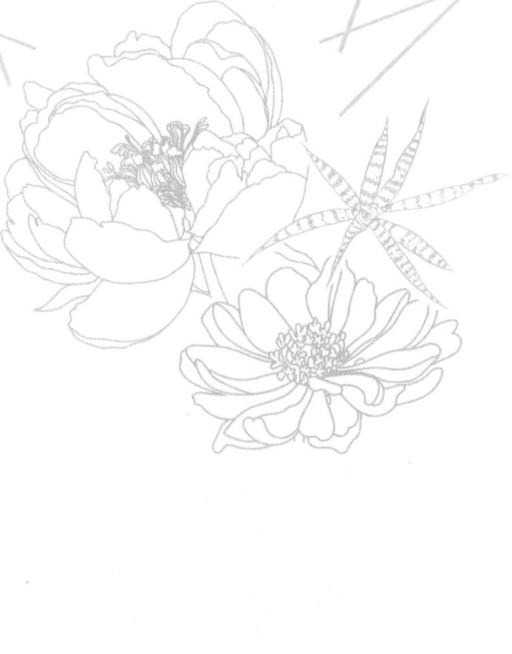

SELF-CARE

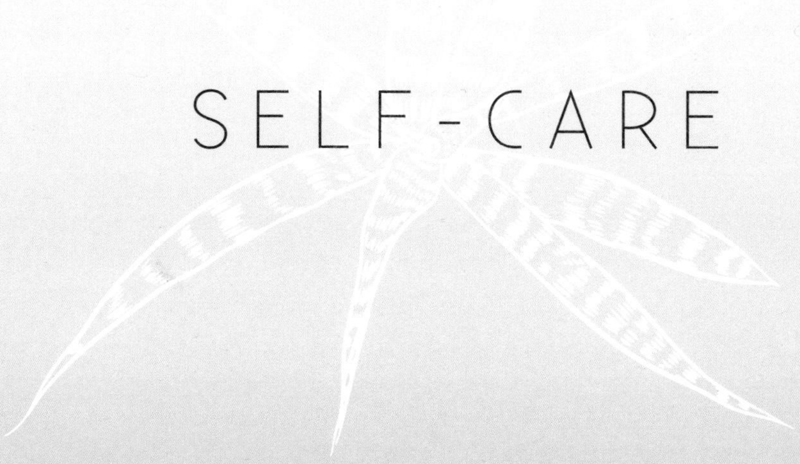

GETTING TO KNOW YOUR INNER SELF IS AN IMPORTANT STEP TOWARD INCREASING YOUR OVERALL HAPPINESS AND WELL-BEING. BY GETTING IN TOUCH WITH HABITS, NEEDS, AND EMOTIONS, AS WELL AS THEIR IMPACT ON YOUR BODY AND MIND, YOU CAN TAKE BETTER CARE OF YOURSELF IN BOTH THE SHORT AND LONG TERM.

Your physical and mental health is shaped by diet, sleep, exercise, and other activities. This journal provides a space for daily observations and reflections on how you spend your time and how you care for yourself. It will help you track the impact of your habits and lifestyle on how you feel physically and mentally in order to find out how to be the healthiest and happiest you can be.

The way you use this journal will depend on your individual lifestyle. You can carry it with you and make notes in real time or reflect back on your day before bed. Savor the chance to get to know yourself better, and cherish the ways you can care for yourself.

RECORD

DATE ___/___/___

AN INTENTION FOR THE DAY:

SLEPT: FROM ___:___ TO ___:___ TOTAL HOURS:___

☐ GOOD DREAMS ☐ BAD DREAMS ☐ NO DREAMS

NOTES:

WHAT I ATE FOR:

BREAKFAST:	LUNCH:
DINNER:	SNACKS:

NUMBER OF CUPS OF WATER I DRANK:___

EXERCISE: ___:___ TO ___:___ MINUTES:___

TYPE:

OTHER ACTIVITIES:

☐ JOURNALING
☐ SOCIAL TIME
☐ MEDITATION
☐ GRATITUDE
☐ TIME OUTSIDE
☐ CREATIVE WORK
☐ SPIRITUAL PRACTICE
☐ SPA DAY
☐ THERAPY
☐ ALONE TIME
☐ BEING SILLY
☐ LEARNING SOMETHING NEW
☐ LISTENING TO MUSIC
☐ COOKING
☐ CLEANING
☐ ___________

REFLECT

PHYSICALLY, I FEEL:

- [ ] ENERGIZED
- [ ] WELL-RESTED
- [ ] STRONG
- [ ] LIMBER
- [ ] RELAXED
- [ ] ______________
- [ ] SLUGGISH
- [ ] TIRED
- [ ] WEAK
- [ ] SORE
- [ ] STRESSED
- [ ] ______________

THINGS THAT WERE FUN OR RELAXING TODAY:

____

____

____

THINGS THAT WERE HARD OR STRESSFUL TODAY:

____

____

____

OTHER THOUGHTS:

____

____

____

____

____

____

____

____

KIND THINGS I DID FOR MYSELF:

____

____

____

TIME:	AS I WOKE UP			AS I WENT TO SLEEP
MOOD:				
NOTES:				

RECORD

DATE ___/___/___

AN INTENTION FOR THE DAY:

SLEPT: FROM ___:___ TO ___:___ TOTAL HOURS: ___

☐ GOOD DREAMS ☐ BAD DREAMS ☐ NO DREAMS

NOTES:

WHAT I ATE FOR:

BREAKFAST:	LUNCH:
DINNER:	SNACKS:

NUMBER OF CUPS OF WATER I DRANK: ___

EXERCISE: ___:___ TO ___:___ MINUTES: ___
TYPE:

OTHER ACTIVITIES:

- ☐ JOURNALING
- ☐ SOCIAL TIME
- ☐ MEDITATION
- ☐ GRATITUDE
- ☐ TIME OUTSIDE
- ☐ CREATIVE WORK
- ☐ SPIRITUAL PRACTICE
- ☐ SPA DAY
- ☐ THERAPY
- ☐ ALONE TIME
- ☐ BEING SILLY
- ☐ LEARNING SOMETHING NEW
- ☐ LISTENING TO MUSIC
- ☐ COOKING
- ☐ CLEANING
- ☐ ___________

REFLECT

PHYSICALLY, I FEEL:

- ☐ ENERGIZED
- ☐ WELL-RESTED
- ☐ STRONG
- ☐ LIMBER
- ☐ RELAXED
- ☐ ____________
- ☐ SLUGGISH
- ☐ TIRED
- ☐ WEAK
- ☐ SORE
- ☐ STRESSED
- ☐ ____________

THINGS THAT WERE FUN OR RELAXING TODAY:

THINGS THAT WERE HARD OR STRESSFUL TODAY:

OTHER THOUGHTS:

KIND THINGS I DID FOR MYSELF:

TIME:	AS I WOKE UP			AS I WENT TO SLEEP
MOOD:				
NOTES:				

RECORD

DATE ___/___/___

AN INTENTION FOR THE DAY:

SLEPT: FROM ___:___ TO ___:___ TOTAL HOURS: ___

☐ GOOD DREAMS ☐ BAD DREAMS ☐ NO DREAMS

NOTES:

WHAT I ATE FOR:

BREAKFAST:	LUNCH:
DINNER:	SNACKS:

NUMBER OF CUPS OF WATER I DRANK: ___

EXERCISE: ___:___ TO ___:___ MINUTES: ___

TYPE:

OTHER ACTIVITIES:

- ☐ JOURNALING
- ☐ SOCIAL TIME
- ☐ MEDITATION
- ☐ GRATITUDE
- ☐ TIME OUTSIDE
- ☐ CREATIVE WORK
- ☐ SPIRITUAL PRACTICE
- ☐ SPA DAY
- ☐ THERAPY
- ☐ ALONE TIME
- ☐ BEING SILLY
- ☐ LEARNING SOMETHING NEW
- ☐ LISTENING TO MUSIC
- ☐ COOKING
- ☐ CLEANING
- ☐ ___

REFLECT

PHYSICALLY, I FEEL:

- [ ] ENERGIZED
- [ ] WELL-RESTED
- [ ] STRONG
- [ ] LIMBER
- [ ] RELAXED
- [ ] ____________
- [ ] SLUGGISH
- [ ] TIRED
- [ ] WEAK
- [ ] SORE
- [ ] STRESSED
- [ ] ____________

THINGS THAT WERE FUN OR RELAXING TODAY:

____

____

____

THINGS THAT WERE HARD OR STRESSFUL TODAY:

____

____

____

OTHER THOUGHTS:

____

____

____

____

____

____

____

____

KIND THINGS I DID FOR MYSELF:

____

____

____

TIME:	AS I WOKE UP			AS I WENT TO SLEEP
MOOD:				
NOTES:				

RECORD

DATE ___/___/___

AN INTENTION FOR THE DAY:

SLEPT: FROM ___:___ TO ___:___ TOTAL HOURS:___

☐ GOOD DREAMS ☐ BAD DREAMS ☐ NO DREAMS

NOTES:

WHAT I ATE FOR:

BREAKFAST:	LUNCH:
DINNER:	SNACKS:

NUMBER OF CUPS OF WATER I DRANK:___

EXERCISE: ___:___ TO ___:___ MINUTES:___

TYPE:

OTHER ACTIVITIES:

- ☐ JOURNALING
- ☐ SOCIAL TIME
- ☐ MEDITATION
- ☐ GRATITUDE
- ☐ TIME OUTSIDE
- ☐ CREATIVE WORK
- ☐ SPIRITUAL PRACTICE
- ☐ SPA DAY
- ☐ THERAPY
- ☐ ALONE TIME
- ☐ BEING SILLY
- ☐ LEARNING SOMETHING NEW
- ☐ LISTENING TO MUSIC
- ☐ COOKING
- ☐ CLEANING
- ☐ ____________

REFLECT

PHYSICALLY, I FEEL:

- ☐ ENERGIZED
- ☐ WELL-RESTED
- ☐ STRONG
- ☐ LIMBER
- ☐ RELAXED
- ☐ ____________
- ☐ SLUGGISH
- ☐ TIRED
- ☐ WEAK
- ☐ SORE
- ☐ STRESSED
- ☐ ____________

THINGS THAT WERE FUN OR RELAXING TODAY:

____

____

____

THINGS THAT WERE HARD OR STRESSFUL TODAY:

____

____

____

OTHER THOUGHTS:

____

____

____

____

____

____

____

____

KIND THINGS I DID FOR MYSELF:

____

____

____

TIME:	AS I WOKE UP			AS I WENT TO SLEEP
MOOD:				
NOTES:				

RECORD

DATE ___/___/___

AN INTENTION FOR THE DAY:

SLEPT: FROM ___:___ TO ___:___ TOTAL HOURS: ___

☐ GOOD DREAMS ☐ BAD DREAMS ☐ NO DREAMS

NOTES:

WHAT I ATE FOR:

BREAKFAST:	LUNCH:
DINNER:	SNACKS:

NUMBER OF CUPS OF WATER I DRANK: ___

EXERCISE: ___:___ TO ___:___ MINUTES: ___

TYPE:

OTHER ACTIVITIES:

- ☐ JOURNALING
- ☐ SOCIAL TIME
- ☐ MEDITATION
- ☐ GRATITUDE
- ☐ TIME OUTSIDE
- ☐ CREATIVE WORK
- ☐ SPIRITUAL PRACTICE
- ☐ SPA DAY
- ☐ THERAPY
- ☐ ALONE TIME
- ☐ BEING SILLY
- ☐ LEARNING SOMETHING NEW
- ☐ LISTENING TO MUSIC
- ☐ COOKING
- ☐ CLEANING
- ☐ __________

REFLECT

PHYSICALLY, I FEEL:

- [ ] ENERGIZED
- [ ] WELL-RESTED
- [ ] STRONG
- [ ] LIMBER
- [ ] RELAXED
- [ ] ______________
- [ ] SLUGGISH
- [ ] TIRED
- [ ] WEAK
- [ ] SORE
- [ ] STRESSED
- [ ] ______________

THINGS THAT WERE FUN OR RELAXING TODAY:

____

____

____

THINGS THAT WERE HARD OR STRESSFUL TODAY:

____

____

____

OTHER THOUGHTS:

____

____

____

____

____

____

____

____

KIND THINGS I DID FOR MYSELF:

____

____

____

TIME:	AS I WOKE UP			AS I WENT TO SLEEP
MOOD:				
NOTES:				

RECORD

DATE ___/___/___

AN INTENTION FOR THE DAY:

SLEPT: FROM ___:___ TO ___:___ TOTAL HOURS:___

☐ GOOD DREAMS ☐ BAD DREAMS ☐ NO DREAMS

NOTES:

WHAT I ATE FOR:

BREAKFAST:	LUNCH:
DINNER:	SNACKS:

NUMBER OF CUPS OF WATER I DRANK:___

EXERCISE: ___:___ TO ___:___ MINUTES:___

TYPE:

OTHER ACTIVITIES:

☐ JOURNALING
☐ SOCIAL TIME
☐ MEDITATION
☐ GRATITUDE
☐ TIME OUTSIDE
☐ CREATIVE WORK
☐ SPIRITUAL PRACTICE
☐ SPA DAY
☐ THERAPY
☐ ALONE TIME
☐ BEING SILLY
☐ LEARNING SOMETHING NEW
☐ LISTENING TO MUSIC
☐ COOKING
☐ CLEANING
☐ ___________

REFLECT

PHYSICALLY, I FEEL:

- ☐ ENERGIZED
- ☐ WELL-RESTED
- ☐ STRONG
- ☐ LIMBER
- ☐ RELAXED
- ☐ ____________
- ☐ SLUGGISH
- ☐ TIRED
- ☐ WEAK
- ☐ SORE
- ☐ STRESSED
- ☐ ____________

THINGS THAT WERE FUN OR RELAXING TODAY:

____

____

____

THINGS THAT WERE HARD OR STRESSFUL TODAY:

____

____

____

OTHER THOUGHTS:

____

____

____

____

____

____

____

____

KIND THINGS I DID FOR MYSELF:

____

____

____

TIME:	AS I WOKE UP			AS I WENT TO SLEEP
MOOD:				
NOTES:				

RECORD

DATE ___/___/___

AN INTENTION FOR THE DAY:

SLEPT: FROM ___:___ TO ___:___ TOTAL HOURS:___

☐ GOOD DREAMS ☐ BAD DREAMS ☐ NO DREAMS

NOTES:

WHAT I ATE FOR:

BREAKFAST:	LUNCH:
DINNER:	SNACKS:

NUMBER OF CUPS OF WATER I DRANK:___

EXERCISE: ___:___ TO ___:___ MINUTES:___
TYPE:

OTHER ACTIVITIES:

- ☐ JOURNALING
- ☐ SOCIAL TIME
- ☐ MEDITATION
- ☐ GRATITUDE
- ☐ TIME OUTSIDE
- ☐ CREATIVE WORK
- ☐ SPIRITUAL PRACTICE
- ☐ SPA DAY
- ☐ THERAPY
- ☐ ALONE TIME
- ☐ BEING SILLY
- ☐ LEARNING SOMETHING NEW
- ☐ LISTENING TO MUSIC
- ☐ COOKING
- ☐ CLEANING
- ☐ ___________

REFLECT

PHYSICALLY, I FEEL:

- ☐ ENERGIZED
- ☐ WELL-RESTED
- ☐ STRONG
- ☐ LIMBER
- ☐ RELAXED
- ☐ ____________
- ☐ SLUGGISH
- ☐ TIRED
- ☐ WEAK
- ☐ SORE
- ☐ STRESSED
- ☐ ____________

THINGS THAT WERE FUN OR RELAXING TODAY:

____

____

____

THINGS THAT WERE HARD OR STRESSFUL TODAY:

____

____

____

OTHER THOUGHTS:

____

____

____

____

____

____

____

____

KIND THINGS I DID FOR MYSELF:

____

____

____

TIME:	AS I WOKE UP			AS I WENT TO SLEEP
MOOD:				
NOTES:				

RECORD

DATE ___/___/___

AN INTENTION FOR THE DAY:

SLEPT: FROM ___:___ TO ___:___ TOTAL HOURS:___

☐ GOOD DREAMS ☐ BAD DREAMS ☐ NO DREAMS

NOTES:

WHAT I ATE FOR:

BREAKFAST:	LUNCH:
DINNER:	SNACKS:

NUMBER OF CUPS OF WATER I DRANK:___

EXERCISE: ___:___ TO ___:___ MINUTES:___

TYPE:

OTHER ACTIVITIES:

- ☐ JOURNALING
- ☐ SOCIAL TIME
- ☐ MEDITATION
- ☐ GRATITUDE
- ☐ TIME OUTSIDE
- ☐ CREATIVE WORK
- ☐ SPIRITUAL PRACTICE
- ☐ SPA DAY
- ☐ THERAPY
- ☐ ALONE TIME
- ☐ BEING SILLY
- ☐ LEARNING SOMETHING NEW
- ☐ LISTENING TO MUSIC
- ☐ COOKING
- ☐ CLEANING
- ☐ ___

REFLECT

PHYSICALLY, I FEEL:

- ☐ ENERGIZED
- ☐ WELL-RESTED
- ☐ STRONG
- ☐ LIMBER
- ☐ RELAXED
- ☐ ______________
- ☐ SLUGGISH
- ☐ TIRED
- ☐ WEAK
- ☐ SORE
- ☐ STRESSED
- ☐ ______________

THINGS THAT WERE FUN OR RELAXING TODAY:

____
____
____

THINGS THAT WERE HARD OR STRESSFUL TODAY:

____
____
____

OTHER THOUGHTS:

____
____
____
____
____
____
____
____

KIND THINGS I DID FOR MYSELF:

____
____
____

TIME:	AS I WOKE UP			AS I WENT TO SLEEP
MOOD:				
NOTES:				

RECORD

DATE ___/___/___

AN INTENTION FOR THE DAY:

SLEPT: FROM ___:___ TO ___:___ TOTAL HOURS:___

☐ GOOD DREAMS ☐ BAD DREAMS ☐ NO DREAMS

NOTES:

WHAT I ATE FOR:

BREAKFAST:	LUNCH:
DINNER:	SNACKS:

NUMBER OF CUPS OF WATER I DRANK:___

EXERCISE: ___:___ TO ___:___ MINUTES:___

TYPE:

OTHER ACTIVITIES:

☐ JOURNALING
☐ SOCIAL TIME
☐ MEDITATION
☐ GRATITUDE
☐ TIME OUTSIDE
☐ CREATIVE WORK
☐ SPIRITUAL PRACTICE
☐ SPA DAY
☐ THERAPY
☐ ALONE TIME
☐ BEING SILLY
☐ LEARNING SOMETHING NEW
☐ LISTENING TO MUSIC
☐ COOKING
☐ CLEANING
☐ ___________

REFLECT

PHYSICALLY, I FEEL:

- [ ] ENERGIZED
- [ ] WELL-RESTED
- [ ] STRONG
- [ ] LIMBER
- [ ] RELAXED
- [ ] ______________
- [ ] SLUGGISH
- [ ] TIRED
- [ ] WEAK
- [ ] SORE
- [ ] STRESSED
- [ ] ______________

THINGS THAT WERE FUN OR RELAXING TODAY:

____
____
____

THINGS THAT WERE HARD OR STRESSFUL TODAY:

____
____
____

OTHER THOUGHTS:

____
____
____
____
____
____
____
____

KIND THINGS I DID FOR MYSELF:

____
____
____

TIME:	AS I WOKE UP			AS I WENT TO SLEEP
MOOD:				
NOTES:				

RECORD

DATE ___/___/___

AN INTENTION FOR THE DAY:

SLEPT: FROM ___:___ TO ___:___ TOTAL HOURS: ___

☐ GOOD DREAMS ☐ BAD DREAMS ☐ NO DREAMS

NOTES:

WHAT I ATE FOR:

BREAKFAST:

LUNCH:

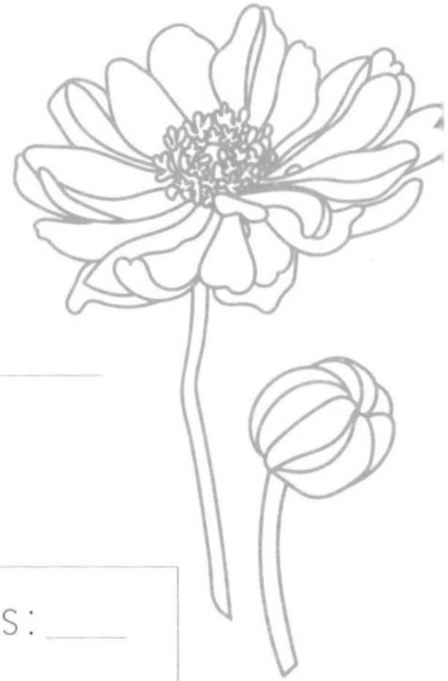

DINNER:

SNACKS:

NUMBER OF CUPS OF WATER I DRANK: ___

EXERCISE: ___:___ TO ___:___ MINUTES: ___

TYPE:

OTHER ACTIVITIES:

☐ JOURNALING
☐ SOCIAL TIME
☐ MEDITATION
☐ GRATITUDE
☐ TIME OUTSIDE
☐ CREATIVE WORK
☐ SPIRITUAL PRACTICE
☐ SPA DAY
☐ THERAPY
☐ ALONE TIME
☐ BEING SILLY
☐ LEARNING SOMETHING NEW
☐ LISTENING TO MUSIC
☐ COOKING
☐ CLEANING
☐ ___________

REFLECT

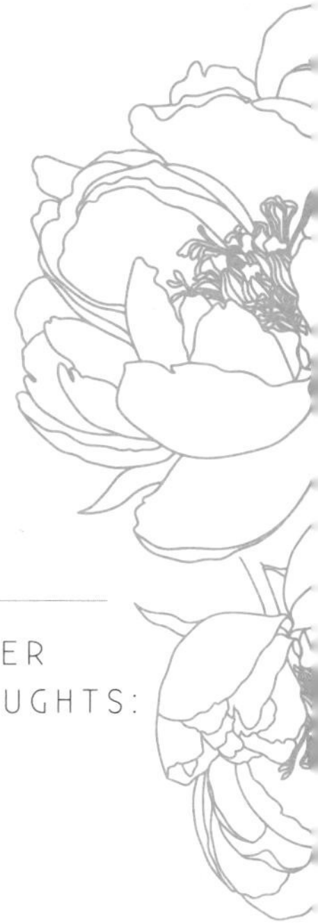

PHYSICALLY, I FEEL:

- ☐ ENERGIZED
- ☐ WELL-RESTED
- ☐ STRONG
- ☐ LIMBER
- ☐ RELAXED
- ☐ ______________
- ☐ SLUGGISH
- ☐ TIRED
- ☐ WEAK
- ☐ SORE
- ☐ STRESSED
- ☐ ______________

THINGS THAT WERE FUN OR RELAXING TODAY:

____

____

____

THINGS THAT WERE HARD OR STRESSFUL TODAY:

____

____

____

OTHER THOUGHTS:

KIND THINGS I DID FOR MYSELF:

____

____

____

TIME:	AS I WOKE UP			AS I WENT TO SLEEP
MOOD:				
NOTES:				

RECORD

DATE ___/___/___

AN INTENTION FOR THE DAY:

SLEPT: FROM ___:___ TO ___:___ TOTAL HOURS:___

☐ GOOD DREAMS ☐ BAD DREAMS ☐ NO DREAMS

NOTES:

WHAT I ATE FOR:

BREAKFAST:	LUNCH:
DINNER:	SNACKS:

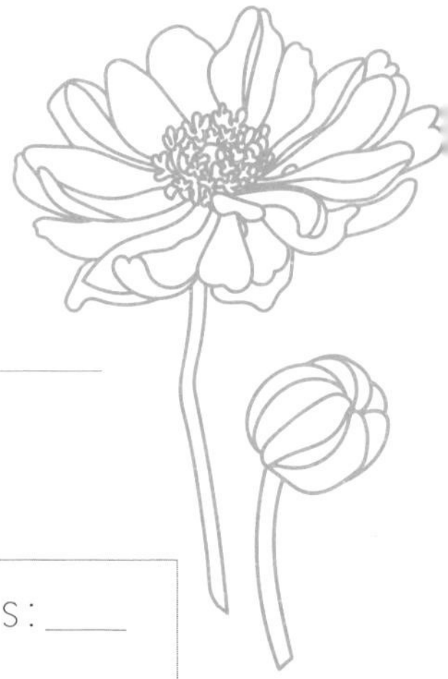

NUMBER OF CUPS OF WATER I DRANK:___

EXERCISE: ___:___ TO ___:___ MINUTES:___

TYPE:

OTHER ACTIVITIES:

- ☐ JOURNALING
- ☐ SOCIAL TIME
- ☐ MEDITATION
- ☐ GRATITUDE
- ☐ TIME OUTSIDE
- ☐ CREATIVE WORK
- ☐ SPIRITUAL PRACTICE
- ☐ SPA DAY
- ☐ THERAPY
- ☐ ALONE TIME
- ☐ BEING SILLY
- ☐ LEARNING SOMETHING NEW
- ☐ LISTENING TO MUSIC
- ☐ COOKING
- ☐ CLEANING
- ☐ ___

REFLECT

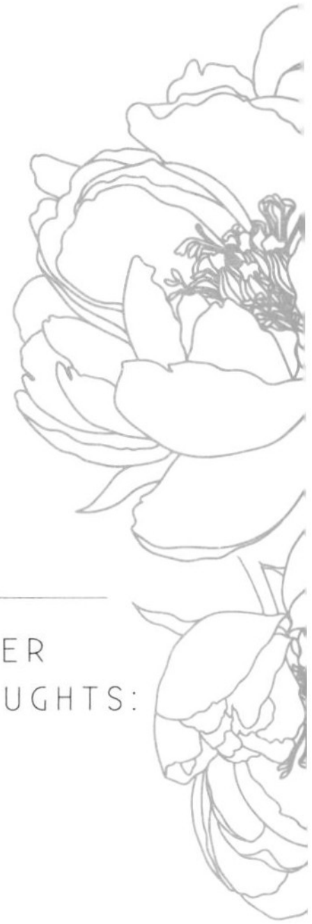

PHYSICALLY, I FEEL:

- ☐ ENERGIZED
- ☐ WELL-RESTED
- ☐ STRONG
- ☐ LIMBER
- ☐ RELAXED
- ☐ ______
- ☐ SLUGGISH
- ☐ TIRED
- ☐ WEAK
- ☐ SORE
- ☐ STRESSED
- ☐ ______

THINGS THAT WERE FUN OR RELAXING TODAY:

THINGS THAT WERE HARD OR STRESSFUL TODAY:

OTHER THOUGHTS:

KIND THINGS I DID FOR MYSELF:

TIME:	AS I WOKE UP			AS I WENT TO SLEEP
MOOD:				
NOTES:				

RECORD

DATE ___/___/___

AN INTENTION FOR THE DAY:

SLEPT: FROM ___ : ___ TO ___ : ___ TOTAL HOURS: ___

☐ GOOD DREAMS ☐ BAD DREAMS ☐ NO DREAMS

NOTES:

WHAT I ATE FOR:

BREAKFAST:

LUNCH:

DINNER:

SNACKS:

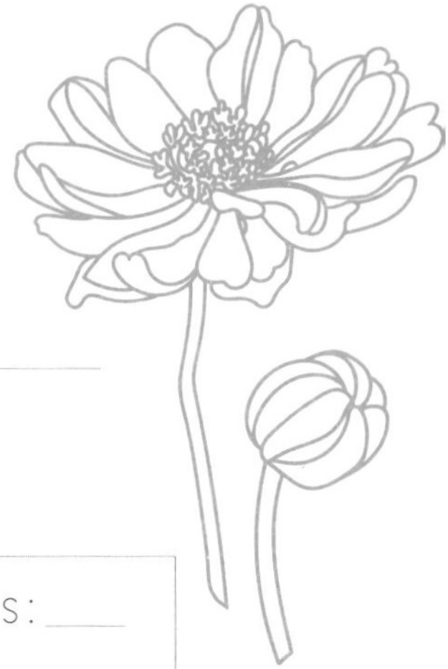

NUMBER OF CUPS OF WATER I DRANK: ___

EXERCISE: ___ : ___ TO ___ : ___ MINUTES: ___

TYPE:

OTHER ACTIVITIES:

☐ JOURNALING
☐ SOCIAL TIME
☐ MEDITATION
☐ GRATITUDE
☐ TIME OUTSIDE
☐ CREATIVE WORK
☐ SPIRITUAL PRACTICE
☐ SPA DAY
☐ THERAPY
☐ ALONE TIME
☐ BEING SILLY
☐ LEARNING SOMETHING NEW
☐ LISTENING TO MUSIC
☐ COOKING
☐ CLEANING
☐ ___

REFLECT

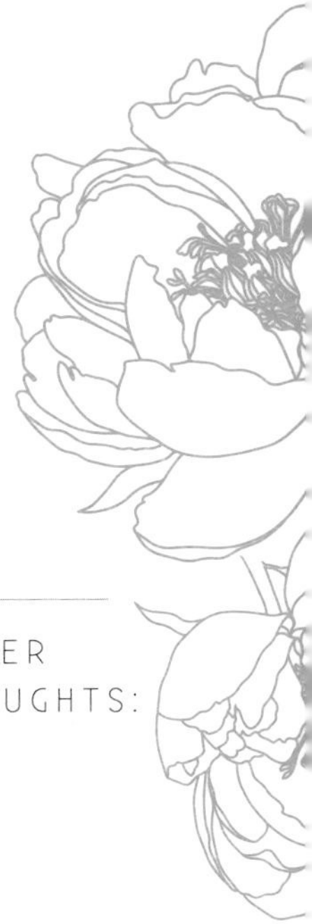

PHYSICALLY, I FEEL:

- [ ] ENERGIZED
- [ ] WELL-RESTED
- [ ] STRONG
- [ ] LIMBER
- [ ] RELAXED
- [ ] ____________
- [ ] SLUGGISH
- [ ] TIRED
- [ ] WEAK
- [ ] SORE
- [ ] STRESSED
- [ ] ____________

THINGS THAT WERE FUN OR RELAXING TODAY:

THINGS THAT WERE HARD OR STRESSFUL TODAY:

OTHER THOUGHTS:

KIND THINGS I DID FOR MYSELF:

TIME:	AS I WOKE UP			AS I WENT TO SLEEP
MOOD:				
NOTES:				

RECORD

DATE ___/___/___

AN INTENTION FOR THE DAY:

SLEPT: FROM ___:___ TO ___:___ TOTAL HOURS:___

☐ GOOD DREAMS ☐ BAD DREAMS ☐ NO DREAMS

NOTES:

WHAT I ATE FOR:

BREAKFAST:	LUNCH:
DINNER:	SNACKS:

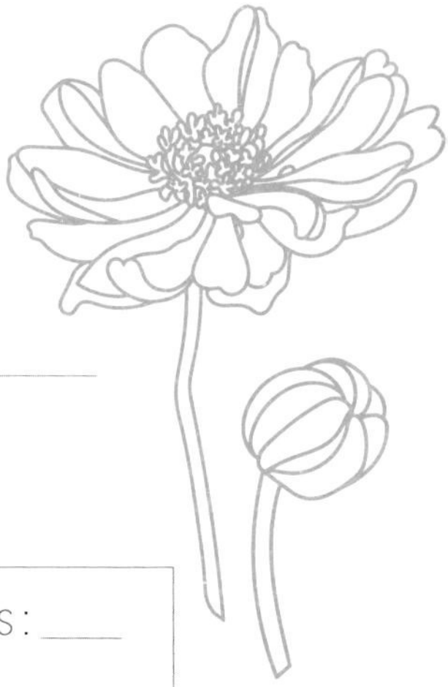

NUMBER OF CUPS OF WATER I DRANK:___

EXERCISE: ___:___ TO ___:___ MINUTES:___

TYPE:

OTHER ACTIVITIES:

☐ JOURNALING
☐ SOCIAL TIME
☐ MEDITATION
☐ GRATITUDE
☐ TIME OUTSIDE
☐ CREATIVE WORK
☐ SPIRITUAL PRACTICE
☐ SPA DAY
☐ THERAPY
☐ ALONE TIME
☐ BEING SILLY
☐ LEARNING SOMETHING NEW
☐ LISTENING TO MUSIC
☐ COOKING
☐ CLEANING
☐ ___

REFLECT

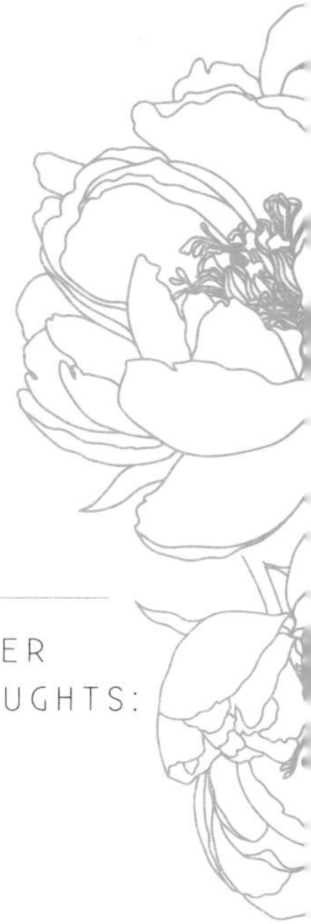

PHYSICALLY, I FEEL:

☐ ENERGIZED	☐ SLUGGISH
☐ WELL-RESTED	☐ TIRED
☐ STRONG	☐ WEAK
☐ LIMBER	☐ SORE
☐ RELAXED	☐ STRESSED
☐ ______________	☐ ______________

THINGS THAT WERE FUN OR RELAXING TODAY:

OTHER THOUGHTS:

THINGS THAT WERE HARD OR STRESSFUL TODAY:

KIND THINGS I DID FOR MYSELF:

TIME:	AS I WOKE UP			AS I WENT TO SLEEP
MOOD:				
NOTES:				

RECORD

DATE ___/___/___

AN INTENTION FOR THE DAY:

SLEPT: FROM ___:___ TO ___:___ TOTAL HOURS:___

☐ GOOD DREAMS ☐ BAD DREAMS ☐ NO DREAMS

NOTES:

WHAT I ATE FOR:

BREAKFAST:

LUNCH:

DINNER:

SNACKS:

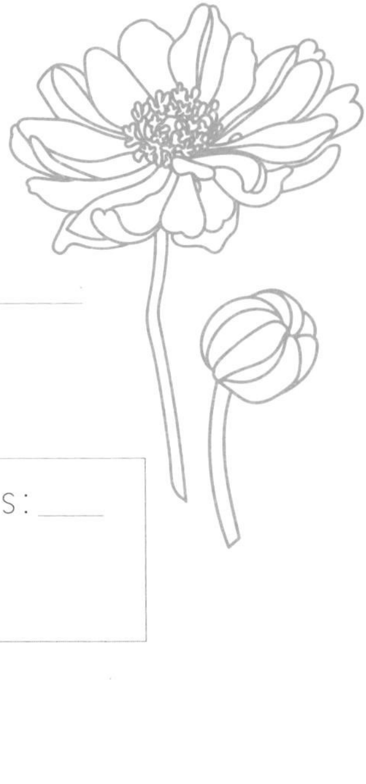

NUMBER OF CUPS OF WATER I DRANK: ___

EXERCISE: ___:___ TO ___:___ MINUTES:___

TYPE:

OTHER ACTIVITIES:

- ☐ JOURNALING
- ☐ SOCIAL TIME
- ☐ MEDITATION
- ☐ GRATITUDE
- ☐ TIME OUTSIDE
- ☐ CREATIVE WORK
- ☐ SPIRITUAL PRACTICE
- ☐ SPA DAY
- ☐ THERAPY
- ☐ ALONE TIME
- ☐ BEING SILLY
- ☐ LEARNING SOMETHING NEW
- ☐ LISTENING TO MUSIC
- ☐ COOKING
- ☐ CLEANING
- ☐ ___

REFLECT

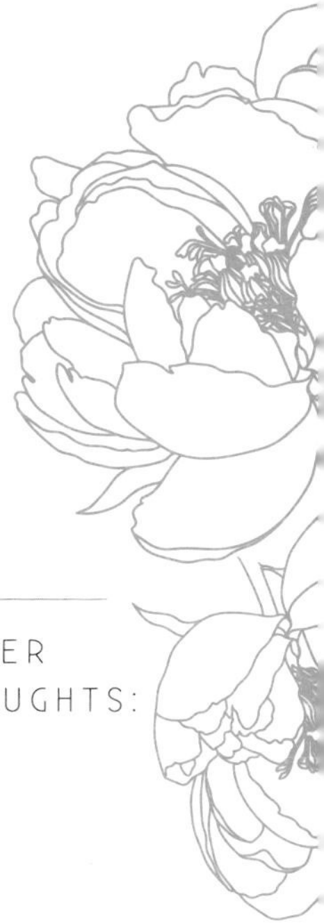

PHYSICALLY, I FEEL:

- ☐ ENERGIZED
- ☐ WELL-RESTED
- ☐ STRONG
- ☐ LIMBER
- ☐ RELAXED
- ☐ ________
- ☐ SLUGGISH
- ☐ TIRED
- ☐ WEAK
- ☐ SORE
- ☐ STRESSED
- ☐ ________

THINGS THAT WERE FUN OR RELAXING TODAY:

____

____

____

THINGS THAT WERE HARD OR STRESSFUL TODAY:

____

____

____

OTHER THOUGHTS:

KIND THINGS I DID FOR MYSELF:

____

____

____

TIME:	AS I WOKE UP			AS I WENT TO SLEEP
MOOD:				
NOTES:				

RECORD

DATE ___/___/___

AN INTENTION FOR THE DAY:

SLEPT: FROM ___:___ TO ___:___ TOTAL HOURS:___

☐ GOOD DREAMS ☐ BAD DREAMS ☐ NO DREAMS

NOTES:

WHAT I ATE FOR:

BREAKFAST:	LUNCH:
DINNER:	SNACKS:

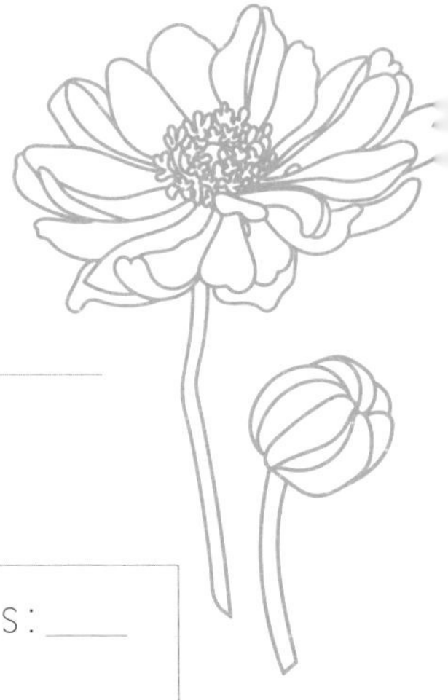

NUMBER OF CUPS OF WATER I DRANK:___

EXERCISE: ___:___ TO ___:___ MINUTES:___
TYPE:

OTHER ACTIVITIES:

- ☐ JOURNALING
- ☐ SOCIAL TIME
- ☐ MEDITATION
- ☐ GRATITUDE
- ☐ TIME OUTSIDE
- ☐ CREATIVE WORK
- ☐ SPIRITUAL PRACTICE
- ☐ SPA DAY
- ☐ THERAPY
- ☐ ALONE TIME
- ☐ BEING SILLY
- ☐ LEARNING SOMETHING NEW
- ☐ LISTENING TO MUSIC
- ☐ COOKING
- ☐ CLEANING
- ☐ ___

REFLECT

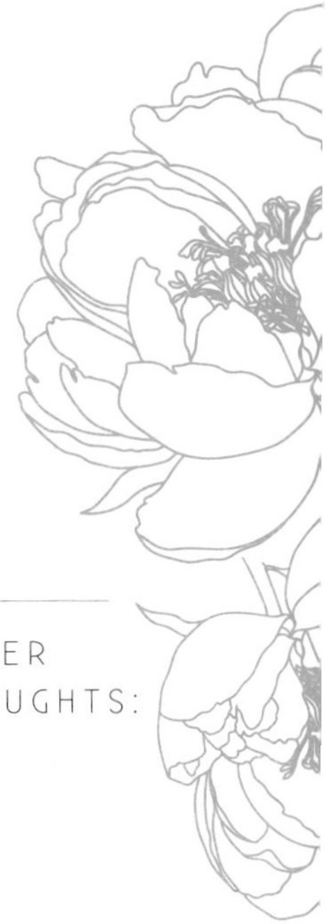

PHYSICALLY, I FEEL:

- [ ] ENERGIZED
- [ ] WELL-RESTED
- [ ] STRONG
- [ ] LIMBER
- [ ] RELAXED
- [ ] ______________
- [ ] SLUGGISH
- [ ] TIRED
- [ ] WEAK
- [ ] SORE
- [ ] STRESSED
- [ ] ______________

THINGS THAT WERE FUN OR RELAXING TODAY:

____

____

____

THINGS THAT WERE HARD OR STRESSFUL TODAY:

____

____

____

OTHER THOUGHTS:

KIND THINGS I DID FOR MYSELF:

____

____

____

TIME:	AS I WOKE UP			AS I WENT TO SLEEP
MOOD:				
NOTES:				

RECORD

DATE ___/___/___

AN INTENTION FOR THE DAY:

SLEPT: FROM ___:___ TO ___:___ TOTAL HOURS: ___

☐ GOOD DREAMS ☐ BAD DREAMS ☐ NO DREAMS

NOTES:

WHAT I ATE FOR:

BREAKFAST:	LUNCH:
DINNER:	SNACKS:

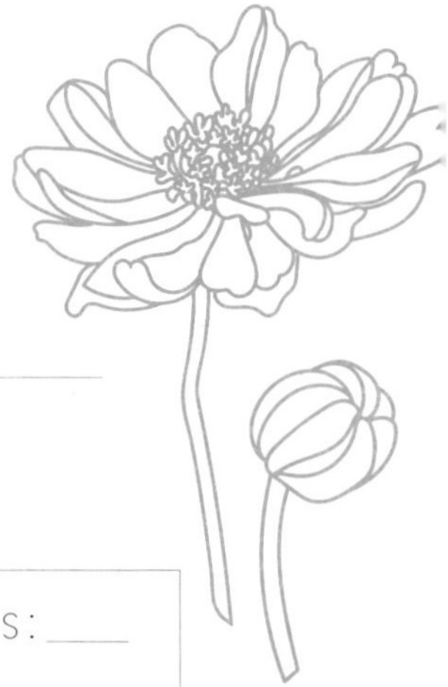

NUMBER OF CUPS OF WATER I DRANK: ___

EXERCISE: ___:___ TO ___:___ MINUTES: ___

TYPE:

OTHER ACTIVITIES:

- ☐ JOURNALING
- ☐ SOCIAL TIME
- ☐ MEDITATION
- ☐ GRATITUDE
- ☐ TIME OUTSIDE
- ☐ CREATIVE WORK
- ☐ SPIRITUAL PRACTICE
- ☐ SPA DAY
- ☐ THERAPY
- ☐ ALONE TIME
- ☐ BEING SILLY
- ☐ LEARNING SOMETHING NEW
- ☐ LISTENING TO MUSIC
- ☐ COOKING
- ☐ CLEANING
- ☐ ___

REFLECT

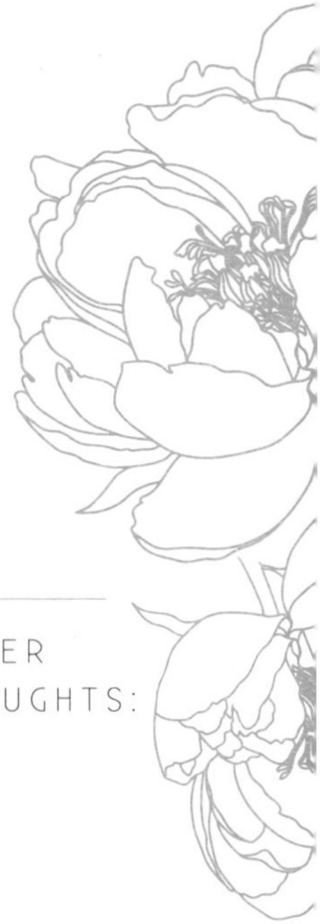

PHYSICALLY, I FEEL:

- [ ] ENERGIZED
- [ ] WELL-RESTED
- [ ] STRONG
- [ ] LIMBER
- [ ] RELAXED
- [ ] ____________________
- [ ] SLUGGISH
- [ ] TIRED
- [ ] WEAK
- [ ] SORE
- [ ] STRESSED
- [ ] ____________________

THINGS THAT WERE FUN OR RELAXING TODAY:

THINGS THAT WERE HARD OR STRESSFUL TODAY:

OTHER THOUGHTS:

KIND THINGS I DID FOR MYSELF:

TIME:	AS I WOKE UP			AS I WENT TO SLEEP
MOOD:				
NOTES:				

RECORD

DATE ___/___/___

AN INTENTION FOR THE DAY:

SLEPT: FROM ___:___ TO ___:___ TOTAL HOURS:___

☐ GOOD DREAMS ☐ BAD DREAMS ☐ NO DREAMS

NOTES:

WHAT I ATE FOR:

BREAKFAST:	LUNCH:
DINNER:	SNACKS:

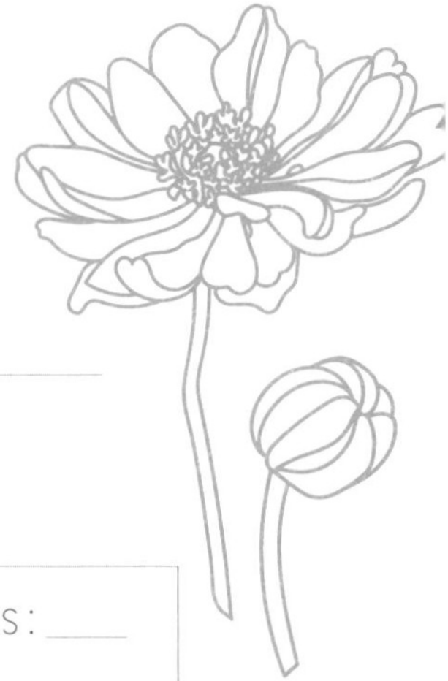

NUMBER OF CUPS OF WATER I DRANK:___

EXERCISE: ___:___ TO ___:___ MINUTES:___

TYPE:

OTHER ACTIVITIES:

☐ JOURNALING
☐ SOCIAL TIME
☐ MEDITATION
☐ GRATITUDE
☐ TIME OUTSIDE
☐ CREATIVE WORK
☐ SPIRITUAL PRACTICE
☐ SPA DAY
☐ THERAPY
☐ ALONE TIME
☐ BEING SILLY
☐ LEARNING SOMETHING NEW
☐ LISTENING TO MUSIC
☐ COOKING
☐ CLEANING
☐ ___

REFLECT

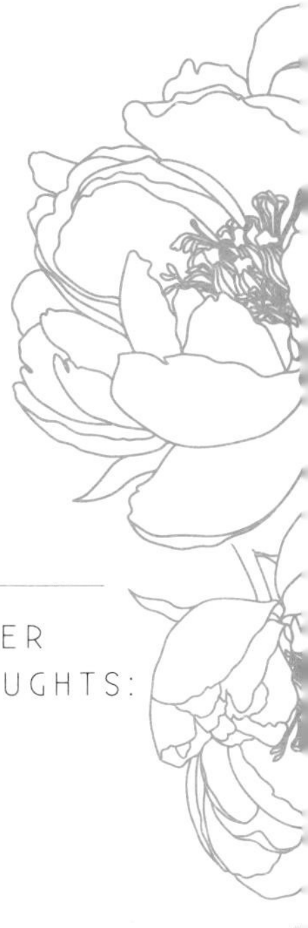

PHYSICALLY, I FEEL:

☐ ENERGIZED	☐ SLUGGISH
☐ WELL-RESTED	☐ TIRED
☐ STRONG	☐ WEAK
☐ LIMBER	☐ SORE
☐ RELAXED	☐ STRESSED
☐ ________	☐ ________

THINGS THAT WERE FUN OR RELAXING TODAY:

THINGS THAT WERE HARD OR STRESSFUL TODAY:

OTHER THOUGHTS:

KIND THINGS I DID FOR MYSELF:

TIME:	AS I WOKE UP			AS I WENT TO SLEEP
MOOD:				
NOTES:				

RECORD

DATE ___/___/___

AN INTENTION FOR THE DAY:

SLEPT: FROM ___:___ TO ___:___ TOTAL HOURS: ___

☐ GOOD DREAMS ☐ BAD DREAMS ☐ NO DREAMS

NOTES:

WHAT I ATE FOR:

BREAKFAST:	LUNCH:
DINNER:	SNACKS:

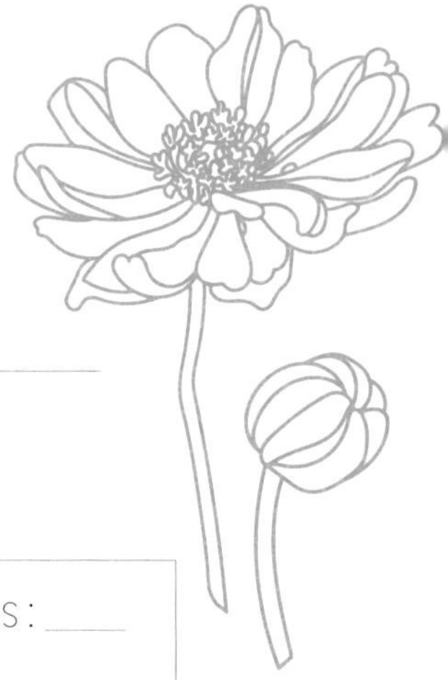

NUMBER OF CUPS OF WATER I DRANK: ___

EXERCISE: ___:___ TO ___:___ MINUTES: ___

TYPE:

OTHER ACTIVITIES:

☐ JOURNALING
☐ SOCIAL TIME
☐ MEDITATION
☐ GRATITUDE
☐ TIME OUTSIDE
☐ CREATIVE WORK
☐ SPIRITUAL PRACTICE
☐ SPA DAY
☐ THERAPY
☐ ALONE TIME
☐ BEING SILLY
☐ LEARNING SOMETHING NEW
☐ LISTENING TO MUSIC
☐ COOKING
☐ CLEANING
☐ ___

REFLECT

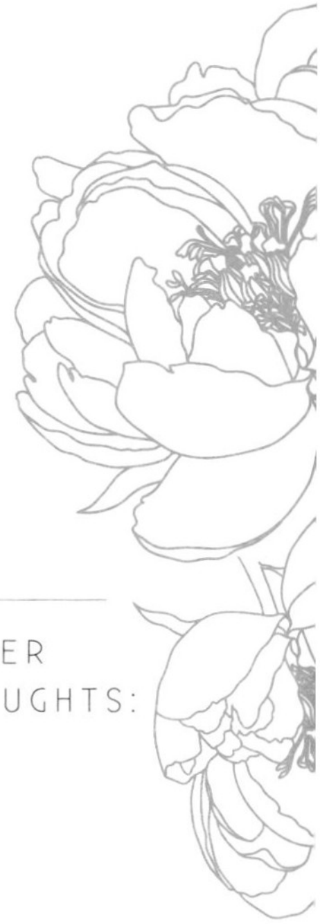

PHYSICALLY, I FEEL:

- ☐ ENERGIZED
- ☐ WELL-RESTED
- ☐ STRONG
- ☐ LIMBER
- ☐ RELAXED
- ☐ ______________
- ☐ SLUGGISH
- ☐ TIRED
- ☐ WEAK
- ☐ SORE
- ☐ STRESSED
- ☐ ______________

THINGS THAT WERE FUN OR RELAXING TODAY:

____

____

____

THINGS THAT WERE HARD OR STRESSFUL TODAY:

____

____

____

OTHER THOUGHTS:

KIND THINGS I DID FOR MYSELF:

____

____

____

TIME:	AS I WOKE UP			AS I WENT TO SLEEP
MOOD:				
NOTES:				

RECORD

DATE ___/___/___

AN INTENTION FOR THE DAY:

SLEPT: FROM ___:___ TO ___:___ TOTAL HOURS: ___

☐ GOOD DREAMS ☐ BAD DREAMS ☐ NO DREAMS

NOTES:

WHAT I ATE FOR:

BREAKFAST:	LUNCH:
DINNER:	SNACKS:

NUMBER OF CUPS OF WATER I DRANK: ___

EXERCISE: ___:___ TO ___:___ MINUTES: ___

TYPE:

OTHER ACTIVITIES:

- ☐ JOURNALING
- ☐ SOCIAL TIME
- ☐ MEDITATION
- ☐ GRATITUDE
- ☐ TIME OUTSIDE
- ☐ CREATIVE WORK
- ☐ SPIRITUAL PRACTICE
- ☐ SPA DAY
- ☐ THERAPY
- ☐ ALONE TIME
- ☐ BEING SILLY
- ☐ LEARNING SOMETHING NEW
- ☐ LISTENING TO MUSIC
- ☐ COOKING
- ☐ CLEANING
- ☐ ___________

REFLECT

PHYSICALLY, I FEEL:

☐ ENERGIZED	☐ SLUGGISH
☐ WELL-RESTED	☐ TIRED
☐ STRONG	☐ WEAK
☐ LIMBER	☐ SORE
☐ RELAXED	☐ STRESSED
☐ ________	☐ ________

THINGS THAT WERE FUN OR RELAXING TODAY:

THINGS THAT WERE HARD OR STRESSFUL TODAY:

OTHER THOUGHTS:

KIND THINGS I DID FOR MYSELF:

TIME:	AS I WOKE UP			AS I WENT TO SLEEP
MOOD:				
NOTES:				

RECORD

DATE ___/___/___

AN INTENTION FOR THE DAY:

SLEPT: FROM ___:___ TO ___:___ TOTAL HOURS:___

☐ GOOD DREAMS ☐ BAD DREAMS ☐ NO DREAMS

NOTES:

WHAT I ATE FOR:

BREAKFAST:	LUNCH:
DINNER:	SNACKS:

NUMBER OF CUPS OF WATER I DRANK:___

EXERCISE: ___:___ TO ___:___ MINUTES:___

TYPE:

OTHER ACTIVITIES:

☐ JOURNALING
☐ SOCIAL TIME
☐ MEDITATION
☐ GRATITUDE
☐ TIME OUTSIDE
☐ CREATIVE WORK
☐ SPIRITUAL PRACTICE
☐ SPA DAY
☐ THERAPY
☐ ALONE TIME
☐ BEING SILLY
☐ LEARNING SOMETHING NEW
☐ LISTENING TO MUSIC
☐ COOKING
☐ CLEANING
☐ ___________

REFLECT

PHYSICALLY, I FEEL:

- ☐ ENERGIZED
- ☐ WELL-RESTED
- ☐ STRONG
- ☐ LIMBER
- ☐ RELAXED
- ☐ ______________
- ☐ SLUGGISH
- ☐ TIRED
- ☐ WEAK
- ☐ SORE
- ☐ STRESSED
- ☐ ______________

THINGS THAT WERE FUN OR RELAXING TODAY:

____

____

____

THINGS THAT WERE HARD OR STRESSFUL TODAY:

____

____

____

OTHER THOUGHTS:

____

____

____

____

____

____

____

____

KIND THINGS I DID FOR MYSELF:

____

____

____

TIME:	AS I WOKE UP			AS I WENT TO SLEEP
MOOD:				
NOTES:				

RECORD

DATE ___/___/___

AN INTENTION FOR THE DAY:

SLEPT: FROM ___:___ TO ___:___ TOTAL HOURS: ___

☐ GOOD DREAMS ☐ BAD DREAMS ☐ NO DREAMS

NOTES:

WHAT I ATE FOR:

BREAKFAST:	LUNCH:
DINNER:	SNACKS:

NUMBER OF CUPS OF WATER I DRANK: ___

EXERCISE: ___:___ TO ___:___ MINUTES: ___

TYPE:

OTHER ACTIVITIES:

- ☐ JOURNALING
- ☐ SOCIAL TIME
- ☐ MEDITATION
- ☐ GRATITUDE
- ☐ TIME OUTSIDE
- ☐ CREATIVE WORK
- ☐ SPIRITUAL PRACTICE
- ☐ SPA DAY
- ☐ THERAPY
- ☐ ALONE TIME
- ☐ BEING SILLY
- ☐ LEARNING SOMETHING NEW
- ☐ LISTENING TO MUSIC
- ☐ COOKING
- ☐ CLEANING
- ☐ ___________

REFLECT

PHYSICALLY, I FEEL:

- ☐ ENERGIZED
- ☐ WELL-RESTED
- ☐ STRONG
- ☐ LIMBER
- ☐ RELAXED
- ☐ ______________
- ☐ SLUGGISH
- ☐ TIRED
- ☐ WEAK
- ☐ SORE
- ☐ STRESSED
- ☐ ______________

THINGS THAT WERE FUN OR RELAXING TODAY:

____

____

____

THINGS THAT WERE HARD OR STRESSFUL TODAY:

____

____

____

OTHER THOUGHTS:

____

____

____

____

____

____

____

____

KIND THINGS I DID FOR MYSELF:

____

____

____

TIME:	AS I WOKE UP			AS I WENT TO SLEEP
MOOD:				
NOTES:				

RECORD

DATE ___/___/___

AN INTENTION FOR THE DAY:

SLEPT: FROM ___:___ TO ___:___ TOTAL HOURS: ___

☐ GOOD DREAMS ☐ BAD DREAMS ☐ NO DREAMS

NOTES:

WHAT I ATE FOR:

BREAKFAST:	LUNCH:
DINNER:	SNACKS:

NUMBER OF CUPS OF WATER I DRANK: ___

EXERCISE: ___:___ TO ___:___ MINUTES: ___

TYPE:

OTHER ACTIVITIES:

- ☐ JOURNALING
- ☐ SOCIAL TIME
- ☐ MEDITATION
- ☐ GRATITUDE
- ☐ TIME OUTSIDE
- ☐ CREATIVE WORK
- ☐ SPIRITUAL PRACTICE
- ☐ SPA DAY
- ☐ THERAPY
- ☐ ALONE TIME
- ☐ BEING SILLY
- ☐ LEARNING SOMETHING NEW
- ☐ LISTENING TO MUSIC
- ☐ COOKING
- ☐ CLEANING
- ☐ ___________

REFLECT

PHYSICALLY, I FEEL:

- ☐ ENERGIZED
- ☐ WELL-RESTED
- ☐ STRONG
- ☐ LIMBER
- ☐ RELAXED
- ☐ ______
- ☐ SLUGGISH
- ☐ TIRED
- ☐ WEAK
- ☐ SORE
- ☐ STRESSED
- ☐ ______

THINGS THAT WERE FUN OR RELAXING TODAY:

THINGS THAT WERE HARD OR STRESSFUL TODAY:

OTHER THOUGHTS:

KIND THINGS I DID FOR MYSELF:

TIME:	AS I WOKE UP			AS I WENT TO SLEEP
MOOD:				
NOTES:				

RECORD

DATE ___/___/___

AN INTENTION FOR THE DAY:

SLEPT: FROM ___:___ TO ___:___ TOTAL HOURS: ___

☐ GOOD DREAMS ☐ BAD DREAMS ☐ NO DREAMS

NOTES:

WHAT I ATE FOR:

BREAKFAST:	LUNCH:
DINNER:	SNACKS:

NUMBER OF CUPS OF WATER I DRANK: ___

EXERCISE: ___:___ TO ___:___ MINUTES: ___

TYPE:

OTHER ACTIVITIES:

- ☐ JOURNALING
- ☐ SOCIAL TIME
- ☐ MEDITATION
- ☐ GRATITUDE
- ☐ TIME OUTSIDE
- ☐ CREATIVE WORK
- ☐ SPIRITUAL PRACTICE
- ☐ SPA DAY
- ☐ THERAPY
- ☐ ALONE TIME
- ☐ BEING SILLY
- ☐ LEARNING SOMETHING NEW
- ☐ LISTENING TO MUSIC
- ☐ COOKING
- ☐ CLEANING
- ☐ __________

REFLECT

PHYSICALLY, I FEEL:

- [ ] ENERGIZED
- [ ] WELL-RESTED
- [ ] STRONG
- [ ] LIMBER
- [ ] RELAXED
- [ ] ______________
- [ ] SLUGGISH
- [ ] TIRED
- [ ] WEAK
- [ ] SORE
- [ ] STRESSED
- [ ] ______________

THINGS THAT WERE FUN OR RELAXING TODAY:

____

____

____

THINGS THAT WERE HARD OR STRESSFUL TODAY:

____

____

____

OTHER THOUGHTS:

____

____

____

____

____

____

____

____

KIND THINGS I DID FOR MYSELF:

____

____

____

TIME:	AS I WOKE UP			AS I WENT TO SLEEP
MOOD:				
NOTES:				

RECORD

DATE ___/___/___

AN INTENTION FOR THE DAY:

SLEPT: FROM ___:___ TO ___:___ TOTAL HOURS:___

☐ GOOD DREAMS ☐ BAD DREAMS ☐ NO DREAMS

NOTES:

WHAT I ATE FOR:

BREAKFAST:	LUNCH:
DINNER:	SNACKS:

NUMBER OF CUPS OF WATER I DRANK:___

EXERCISE: ___:___ TO ___:___ MINUTES:___

TYPE:

OTHER ACTIVITIES:

- ☐ JOURNALING
- ☐ SOCIAL TIME
- ☐ MEDITATION
- ☐ GRATITUDE
- ☐ TIME OUTSIDE
- ☐ CREATIVE WORK
- ☐ SPIRITUAL PRACTICE
- ☐ SPA DAY
- ☐ THERAPY
- ☐ ALONE TIME
- ☐ BEING SILLY
- ☐ LEARNING SOMETHING NEW
- ☐ LISTENING TO MUSIC
- ☐ COOKING
- ☐ CLEANING
- ☐ ___________

REFLECT

PHYSICALLY, I FEEL:

- ☐ ENERGIZED
- ☐ WELL-RESTED
- ☐ STRONG
- ☐ LIMBER
- ☐ RELAXED
- ☐ ____________
- ☐ SLUGGISH
- ☐ TIRED
- ☐ WEAK
- ☐ SORE
- ☐ STRESSED
- ☐ ____________

THINGS THAT WERE FUN OR RELAXING TODAY:

____

____

____

THINGS THAT WERE HARD OR STRESSFUL TODAY:

____

____

____

OTHER THOUGHTS:

____

____

____

____

____

____

____

____

KIND THINGS I DID FOR MYSELF:

____

____

____

TIME:	AS I WOKE UP			AS I WENT TO SLEEP
MOOD:				
NOTES:				

RECORD

DATE ___/___/___

AN INTENTION FOR THE DAY:

SLEPT: FROM ____:____ TO ____:____ TOTAL HOURS:____

☐ GOOD DREAMS ☐ BAD DREAMS ☐ NO DREAMS

NOTES:

WHAT I ATE FOR:

BREAKFAST:	LUNCH:
DINNER:	SNACKS:

NUMBER OF CUPS OF WATER I DRANK:____

EXERCISE: ____:____ TO ____:____ MINUTES:____

TYPE:

OTHER ACTIVITIES:

- ☐ JOURNALING
- ☐ SOCIAL TIME
- ☐ MEDITATION
- ☐ GRATITUDE
- ☐ TIME OUTSIDE
- ☐ CREATIVE WORK
- ☐ SPIRITUAL PRACTICE
- ☐ SPA DAY
- ☐ THERAPY
- ☐ ALONE TIME
- ☐ BEING SILLY
- ☐ LEARNING SOMETHING NEW
- ☐ LISTENING TO MUSIC
- ☐ COOKING
- ☐ CLEANING
- ☐ ____________

REFLECT

PHYSICALLY, I FEEL:

- [ ] ENERGIZED
- [ ] WELL-RESTED
- [ ] STRONG
- [ ] LIMBER
- [ ] RELAXED
- [ ] ______________

- [ ] SLUGGISH
- [ ] TIRED
- [ ] WEAK
- [ ] SORE
- [ ] STRESSED
- [ ] ______________

THINGS THAT WERE FUN OR RELAXING TODAY:

____
____
____

THINGS THAT WERE HARD OR STRESSFUL TODAY:

____
____
____

OTHER THOUGHTS:

____
____
____
____
____
____
____
____

KIND THINGS I DID FOR MYSELF:

____
____
____

TIME:	AS I WOKE UP			AS I WENT TO SLEEP
MOOD:				
NOTES:				

RECORD

DATE ___/___/___

AN INTENTION FOR THE DAY:

SLEPT: FROM ___:___ TO ___:___ TOTAL HOURS: ___

☐ GOOD DREAMS ☐ BAD DREAMS ☐ NO DREAMS

NOTES:

WHAT I ATE FOR:

BREAKFAST:	LUNCH:
DINNER:	SNACKS:

NUMBER OF CUPS OF WATER I DRANK: ___

EXERCISE: ___:___ TO ___:___ MINUTES: ___

TYPE:

OTHER ACTIVITIES:

- ☐ JOURNALING
- ☐ SOCIAL TIME
- ☐ MEDITATION
- ☐ GRATITUDE
- ☐ TIME OUTSIDE
- ☐ CREATIVE WORK
- ☐ SPIRITUAL PRACTICE
- ☐ SPA DAY
- ☐ THERAPY
- ☐ ALONE TIME
- ☐ BEING SILLY
- ☐ LEARNING SOMETHING NEW
- ☐ LISTENING TO MUSIC
- ☐ COOKING
- ☐ CLEANING
- ☐ ________

REFLECT

PHYSICALLY, I FEEL:

- [ ] ENERGIZED
- [ ] WELL-RESTED
- [ ] STRONG
- [ ] LIMBER
- [ ] RELAXED
- [ ] ________
- [ ] SLUGGISH
- [ ] TIRED
- [ ] WEAK
- [ ] SORE
- [ ] STRESSED
- [ ] ________

THINGS THAT WERE FUN OR RELAXING TODAY:

THINGS THAT WERE HARD OR STRESSFUL TODAY:

OTHER THOUGHTS:

KIND THINGS I DID FOR MYSELF:

TIME:	AS I WOKE UP			AS I WENT TO SLEEP
MOOD:				
NOTES:				

RECORD

DATE ___/___/___

AN INTENTION FOR THE DAY:

SLEPT: FROM ___:___ TO ___:___ TOTAL HOURS: ___

☐ GOOD DREAMS ☐ BAD DREAMS ☐ NO DREAMS

NOTES:

WHAT I ATE FOR:

BREAKFAST:	LUNCH:
DINNER:	SNACKS:

NUMBER OF CUPS OF WATER I DRANK: ___

EXERCISE: ___:___ TO ___:___ MINUTES: ___
TYPE:

OTHER ACTIVITIES:

- ☐ JOURNALING
- ☐ SOCIAL TIME
- ☐ MEDITATION
- ☐ GRATITUDE
- ☐ TIME OUTSIDE
- ☐ CREATIVE WORK
- ☐ SPIRITUAL PRACTICE
- ☐ SPA DAY
- ☐ THERAPY
- ☐ ALONE TIME
- ☐ BEING SILLY
- ☐ LEARNING SOMETHING NEW
- ☐ LISTENING TO MUSIC
- ☐ COOKING
- ☐ CLEANING
- ☐ ___________

REFLECT

PHYSICALLY, I FEEL:

- ☐ ENERGIZED
- ☐ WELL-RESTED
- ☐ STRONG
- ☐ LIMBER
- ☐ RELAXED
- ☐ ______
- ☐ SLUGGISH
- ☐ TIRED
- ☐ WEAK
- ☐ SORE
- ☐ STRESSED
- ☐ ______

THINGS THAT WERE FUN OR RELAXING TODAY:

______

______

______

THINGS THAT WERE HARD OR STRESSFUL TODAY:

______

______

______

OTHER THOUGHTS:

______

______

______

______

______

______

______

______

KIND THINGS I DID FOR MYSELF:

______

______

______

TIME:	AS I WOKE UP			AS I WENT TO SLEEP
MOOD:				
NOTES:				

RECORD

DATE ___/___/___

AN INTENTION FOR THE DAY:

SLEPT: FROM ___:___ TO ___:___ TOTAL HOURS: ___

☐ GOOD DREAMS ☐ BAD DREAMS ☐ NO DREAMS

NOTES:

WHAT I ATE FOR:

BREAKFAST:	LUNCH:
DINNER:	SNACKS:

NUMBER OF CUPS OF WATER I DRANK: ___

EXERCISE: ___:___ TO ___:___ TOTAL MINUTES: ___

TYPE:

OTHER ACTIVITIES:

- ☐ JOURNALING
- ☐ SOCIAL TIME
- ☐ MEDITATION
- ☐ GRATITUDE
- ☐ TIME OUTSIDE
- ☐ CREATIVE WORK
- ☐ SPIRITUAL PRACTICE
- ☐ SPA DAY
- ☐ THERAPY
- ☐ ALONE TIME
- ☐ BEING SILLY
- ☐ LEARNING SOMETHING NEW
- ☐ LISTENING TO MUSIC
- ☐ COOKING
- ☐ CLEANING
- ☐ ___________

REFLECT

PHYSICALLY, I FEEL:

☐ ENERGIZED	☐ SLUGGISH
☐ WELL-RESTED	☐ TIRED
☐ STRONG	☐ WEAK
☐ LIMBER	☐ SORE
☐ RELAXED	☐ STRESSED
☐ ______________	☐ ______________

THINGS THAT WERE FUN OR RELAXING TODAY:

____

____

____

THINGS THAT WERE HARD OR STRESSFUL TODAY:

____

____

____

OTHER THOUGHTS:

____

____

____

____

____

____

____

____

KIND THINGS I DID FOR MYSELF:

____

____

____

TIME:	AS I WOKE UP			AS I WENT TO SLEEP
MOOD:				
NOTES:				

RECORD

DATE ___/___/___

AN INTENTION FOR THE DAY:

SLEPT: FROM ___:___ TO ___:___ TOTAL HOURS: ___

☐ GOOD DREAMS ☐ BAD DREAMS ☐ NO DREAMS

NOTES:

WHAT I ATE FOR:

BREAKFAST:	LUNCH:
DINNER:	SNACKS:

NUMBER OF CUPS OF WATER I DRANK: ___

EXERCISE: ___:___ TO ___:___ TOTAL MINUTES: ___

TYPE:

OTHER ACTIVITIES:

- ☐ JOURNALING
- ☐ SOCIAL TIME
- ☐ MEDITATION
- ☐ GRATITUDE
- ☐ TIME OUTSIDE
- ☐ CREATIVE WORK
- ☐ SPIRITUAL PRACTICE
- ☐ SPA DAY
- ☐ THERAPY
- ☐ ALONE TIME
- ☐ BEING SILLY
- ☐ LEARNING SOMETHING NEW
- ☐ LISTENING TO MUSIC
- ☐ COOKING
- ☐ CLEANING
- ☐ __________

REFLECT

PHYSICALLY, I FEEL:

- [ ] ENERGIZED
- [ ] WELL-RESTED
- [ ] STRONG
- [ ] LIMBER
- [ ] RELAXED
- [ ] ____________
- [ ] SLUGGISH
- [ ] TIRED
- [ ] WEAK
- [ ] SORE
- [ ] STRESSED
- [ ] ____________

THINGS THAT WERE FUN OR RELAXING TODAY:

____

____

____

THINGS THAT WERE HARD OR STRESSFUL TODAY:

____

____

____

OTHER THOUGHTS:

____

____

____

____

____

____

____

____

KIND THINGS I DID FOR MYSELF:

____

____

____

TIME:	AS I WOKE UP			AS I WENT TO SLEEP
MOOD:				
NOTES:				

RECORD

DATE ___/___/___

AN INTENTION FOR THE DAY:

SLEPT: FROM ___:___ TO ___:___ TOTAL HOURS: ___

☐ GOOD DREAMS ☐ BAD DREAMS ☐ NO DREAMS

NOTES:

WHAT I ATE FOR:

BREAKFAST:	LUNCH:
DINNER:	SNACKS:

NUMBER OF CUPS OF WATER I DRANK: ___

EXERCISE: ___:___ TO ___:___ TOTAL MINUTES: ___

TYPE:

OTHER ACTIVITIES:

- ☐ JOURNALING
- ☐ SOCIAL TIME
- ☐ MEDITATION
- ☐ GRATITUDE
- ☐ TIME OUTSIDE
- ☐ CREATIVE WORK
- ☐ SPIRITUAL PRACTICE
- ☐ SPA DAY
- ☐ THERAPY
- ☐ ALONE TIME
- ☐ BEING SILLY
- ☐ LEARNING SOMETHING NEW
- ☐ LISTENING TO MUSIC
- ☐ COOKING
- ☐ CLEANING
- ☐ ___

REFLECT

PHYSICALLY, I FEEL:

- [ ] ENERGIZED
- [ ] WELL-RESTED
- [ ] STRONG
- [ ] LIMBER
- [ ] RELAXED
- [ ] ______________
- [ ] SLUGGISH
- [ ] TIRED
- [ ] WEAK
- [ ] SORE
- [ ] STRESSED
- [ ] ______________

THINGS THAT WERE FUN OR RELAXING TODAY:

____

____

____

THINGS THAT WERE HARD OR STRESSFUL TODAY:

____

____

____

OTHER THOUGHTS:

____

____

____

____

____

____

____

____

KIND THINGS I DID FOR MYSELF:

____

____

____

TIME:	AS I WOKE UP			AS I WENT TO SLEEP
MOOD:				
NOTES:				

RECORD

DATE ___/___/___

AN INTENTION FOR THE DAY:

SLEPT: FROM ___:___ TO ___:___ TOTAL HOURS:___

☐ GOOD DREAMS ☐ BAD DREAMS ☐ NO DREAMS

NOTES:

WHAT I ATE FOR:

BREAKFAST:	LUNCH:
DINNER:	SNACKS:

NUMBER OF CUPS OF WATER I DRANK:___

EXERCISE: ___:___ TO ___:___ TOTAL MINUTES:___

TYPE:

OTHER ACTIVITIES:

- ☐ JOURNALING
- ☐ SOCIAL TIME
- ☐ MEDITATION
- ☐ GRATITUDE
- ☐ TIME OUTSIDE
- ☐ CREATIVE WORK
- ☐ SPIRITUAL PRACTICE
- ☐ SPA DAY
- ☐ THERAPY
- ☐ ALONE TIME
- ☐ BEING SILLY
- ☐ LEARNING SOMETHING NEW
- ☐ LISTENING TO MUSIC
- ☐ COOKING
- ☐ CLEANING
- ☐ ___________

REFLECT

PHYSICALLY, I FEEL:

- [ ] ENERGIZED
- [ ] WELL-RESTED
- [ ] STRONG
- [ ] LIMBER
- [ ] RELAXED
- [ ] ______________
- [ ] SLUGGISH
- [ ] TIRED
- [ ] WEAK
- [ ] SORE
- [ ] STRESSED
- [ ] ______________

THINGS THAT WERE FUN OR RELAXING TODAY:

____

____

____

THINGS THAT WERE HARD OR STRESSFUL TODAY:

____

____

____

OTHER THOUGHTS:

____

____

____

____

____

____

____

____

KIND THINGS I DID FOR MYSELF:

____

____

____

TIME:	AS I WOKE UP			AS I WENT TO SLEEP
MOOD:				
NOTES:				

RECORD

DATE ___/___/___

AN INTENTION FOR THE DAY:

SLEPT: FROM ___:___ TO ___:___ TOTAL HOURS:___

☐ GOOD DREAMS ☐ BAD DREAMS ☐ NO DREAMS

NOTES:

WHAT I ATE FOR:

BREAKFAST:	LUNCH:
DINNER:	SNACKS:

NUMBER OF CUPS OF WATER I DRANK:___

EXERCISE: ___:___ TO ___:___ TOTAL MINUTES:___

TYPE:

OTHER ACTIVITIES:

- ☐ JOURNALING
- ☐ SOCIAL TIME
- ☐ MEDITATION
- ☐ GRATITUDE
- ☐ TIME OUTSIDE
- ☐ CREATIVE WORK
- ☐ SPIRITUAL PRACTICE
- ☐ SPA DAY
- ☐ THERAPY
- ☐ ALONE TIME
- ☐ BEING SILLY
- ☐ LEARNING SOMETHING NEW
- ☐ LISTENING TO MUSIC
- ☐ COOKING
- ☐ CLEANING
- ☐ ___________

REFLECT

PHYSICALLY, I FEEL:

- [ ] ENERGIZED
- [ ] WELL-RESTED
- [ ] STRONG
- [ ] LIMBER
- [ ] RELAXED
- [ ] ______________
- [ ] SLUGGISH
- [ ] TIRED
- [ ] WEAK
- [ ] SORE
- [ ] STRESSED
- [ ] ______________

THINGS THAT WERE FUN OR RELAXING TODAY:

____

____

____

THINGS THAT WERE HARD OR STRESSFUL TODAY:

____

____

____

OTHER THOUGHTS:

____

____

____

____

____

____

____

____

KIND THINGS I DID FOR MYSELF:

____

____

____

TIME:	AS I WOKE UP			AS I WENT TO SLEEP
MOOD:				
NOTES:				

RECORD

DATE ___/___/___

AN INTENTION FOR THE DAY:

SLEPT: FROM ___:___ TO ___:___ TOTAL HOURS:___

☐ GOOD DREAMS ☐ BAD DREAMS ☐ NO DREAMS

NOTES:

WHAT I ATE FOR:

BREAKFAST:	LUNCH:
DINNER:	SNACKS:

NUMBER OF CUPS OF WATER I DRANK:___

EXERCISE: ___:___ TO ___:___ TOTAL MINUTES:___

TYPE:

OTHER ACTIVITIES:

- ☐ JOURNALING
- ☐ SOCIAL TIME
- ☐ MEDITATION
- ☐ GRATITUDE
- ☐ TIME OUTSIDE
- ☐ CREATIVE WORK
- ☐ SPIRITUAL PRACTICE
- ☐ SPA DAY
- ☐ THERAPY
- ☐ ALONE TIME
- ☐ BEING SILLY
- ☐ LEARNING SOMETHING NEW
- ☐ LISTENING TO MUSIC
- ☐ COOKING
- ☐ CLEANING
- ☐ ___________

REFLECT

PHYSICALLY, I FEEL:

- ☐ ENERGIZED
- ☐ WELL-RESTED
- ☐ STRONG
- ☐ LIMBER
- ☐ RELAXED
- ☐ ____________
- ☐ SLUGGISH
- ☐ TIRED
- ☐ WEAK
- ☐ SORE
- ☐ STRESSED
- ☐ ____________

THINGS THAT WERE FUN OR RELAXING TODAY:

____

____

____

THINGS THAT WERE HARD OR STRESSFUL TODAY:

____

____

____

OTHER THOUGHTS:

____

____

____

____

____

____

____

____

KIND THINGS I DID FOR MYSELF:

____

____

____

TIME:	AS I WOKE UP			AS I WENT TO SLEEP
MOOD:				
NOTES:				

RECORD

DATE ____/____/____

AN INTENTION FOR THE DAY:

SLEPT: FROM ____:____ TO ____:____ TOTAL HOURS:____

☐ GOOD DREAMS ☐ BAD DREAMS ☐ NO DREAMS

NOTES:

WHAT I ATE FOR:

BREAKFAST:	LUNCH:
DINNER:	SNACKS:

NUMBER OF CUPS OF WATER I DRANK:____

EXERCISE: ____:____ TO ____:____ TOTAL MINUTES:____
TYPE:

OTHER ACTIVITIES:

- ☐ JOURNALING
- ☐ SOCIAL TIME
- ☐ MEDITATION
- ☐ GRATITUDE
- ☐ TIME OUTSIDE
- ☐ CREATIVE WORK
- ☐ SPIRITUAL PRACTICE
- ☐ SPA DAY
- ☐ THERAPY
- ☐ ALONE TIME
- ☐ BEING SILLY
- ☐ LEARNING SOMETHING NEW
- ☐ LISTENING TO MUSIC
- ☐ COOKING
- ☐ CLEANING
- ☐ ____________

REFLECT

PHYSICALLY, I FEEL:

- [ ] ENERGIZED
- [ ] WELL-RESTED
- [ ] STRONG
- [ ] LIMBER
- [ ] RELAXED
- [ ] ____________
- [ ] SLUGGISH
- [ ] TIRED
- [ ] WEAK
- [ ] SORE
- [ ] STRESSED
- [ ] ____________

THINGS THAT WERE FUN OR RELAXING TODAY:

____

____

____

THINGS THAT WERE HARD OR STRESSFUL TODAY:

____

____

____

OTHER THOUGHTS:

____

____

____

____

____

____

____

____

KIND THINGS I DID FOR MYSELF:

____

____

____

TIME:	AS I WOKE UP			AS I WENT TO SLEEP
MOOD:				
NOTES:				

RECORD

DATE ___/___/___

AN INTENTION FOR THE DAY:

SLEPT: FROM ___:___ TO ___:___ TOTAL HOURS:___

☐ GOOD DREAMS ☐ BAD DREAMS ☐ NO DREAMS

NOTES:

WHAT I ATE FOR:

BREAKFAST:	LUNCH:
DINNER:	SNACKS:

NUMBER OF CUPS OF WATER I DRANK: ___

EXERCISE: ___:___ TO ___:___ TOTAL MINUTES:___

TYPE:

OTHER ACTIVITIES:

- ☐ JOURNALING
- ☐ SOCIAL TIME
- ☐ MEDITATION
- ☐ GRATITUDE
- ☐ TIME OUTSIDE
- ☐ CREATIVE WORK
- ☐ SPIRITUAL PRACTICE
- ☐ SPA DAY
- ☐ THERAPY
- ☐ ALONE TIME
- ☐ BEING SILLY
- ☐ LEARNING SOMETHING NEW
- ☐ LISTENING TO MUSIC
- ☐ COOKING
- ☐ CLEANING
- ☐ ___________

REFLECT

PHYSICALLY, I FEEL:

- ☐ ENERGIZED
- ☐ WELL-RESTED
- ☐ STRONG
- ☐ LIMBER
- ☐ RELAXED
- ☐ ____________
- ☐ SLUGGISH
- ☐ TIRED
- ☐ WEAK
- ☐ SORE
- ☐ STRESSED
- ☐ ____________

THINGS THAT WERE FUN OR RELAXING TODAY:

____

____

____

THINGS THAT WERE HARD OR STRESSFUL TODAY:

____

____

____

OTHER THOUGHTS:

____

____

____

____

____

____

____

____

KIND THINGS I DID FOR MYSELF:

____

____

____

TIME:	AS I WOKE UP			AS I WENT TO SLEEP
MOOD:				
NOTES:				

RECORD

DATE ___/___/___

AN INTENTION FOR THE DAY:

SLEPT: FROM ___:___ TO ___:___ TOTAL HOURS:___

☐ GOOD DREAMS ☐ BAD DREAMS ☐ NO DREAMS

NOTES:

WHAT I ATE FOR:

BREAKFAST:	LUNCH:
DINNER:	SNACKS:

NUMBER OF CUPS OF WATER I DRANK:___

EXERCISE: ___:___ TO ___:___ TOTAL MINUTES:___

TYPE:

OTHER ACTIVITIES:

- ☐ JOURNALING
- ☐ SOCIAL TIME
- ☐ MEDITATION
- ☐ GRATITUDE
- ☐ TIME OUTSIDE
- ☐ CREATIVE WORK
- ☐ SPIRITUAL PRACTICE
- ☐ SPA DAY
- ☐ THERAPY
- ☐ ALONE TIME
- ☐ BEING SILLY
- ☐ LEARNING SOMETHING NEW
- ☐ LISTENING TO MUSIC
- ☐ COOKING
- ☐ CLEANING
- ☐ ___________

REFLECT

PHYSICALLY, I FEEL:

- [ ] ENERGIZED
- [ ] WELL-RESTED
- [ ] STRONG
- [ ] LIMBER
- [ ] RELAXED
- [ ] ______________
- [ ] SLUGGISH
- [ ] TIRED
- [ ] WEAK
- [ ] SORE
- [ ] STRESSED
- [ ] ______________

THINGS THAT WERE FUN OR RELAXING TODAY:

____

____

____

THINGS THAT WERE HARD OR STRESSFUL TODAY:

____

____

____

OTHER THOUGHTS:

____

____

____

____

____

____

____

____

KIND THINGS I DID FOR MYSELF:

____

____

____

TIME:	AS I WOKE UP			AS I WENT TO SLEEP
MOOD:				
NOTES:				

RECORD

DATE ___/___/___

AN INTENTION FOR THE DAY:

SLEPT: FROM ___:___ TO ___:___ TOTAL HOURS:___

☐ GOOD DREAMS ☐ BAD DREAMS ☐ NO DREAMS

NOTES:

WHAT I ATE FOR:

BREAKFAST:	LUNCH:
DINNER:	SNACKS:

NUMBER OF CUPS OF WATER I DRANK:___

EXERCISE: ___:___ TO ___:___ TOTAL MINUTES:___

TYPE:

OTHER ACTIVITIES:

- ☐ JOURNALING
- ☐ SOCIAL TIME
- ☐ MEDITATION
- ☐ GRATITUDE
- ☐ TIME OUTSIDE
- ☐ CREATIVE WORK
- ☐ SPIRITUAL PRACTICE
- ☐ SPA DAY
- ☐ THERAPY
- ☐ ALONE TIME
- ☐ BEING SILLY
- ☐ LEARNING SOMETHING NEW
- ☐ LISTENING TO MUSIC
- ☐ COOKING
- ☐ CLEANING
- ☐ ___________

REFLECT

PHYSICALLY, I FEEL:

- ☐ ENERGIZED
- ☐ WELL-RESTED
- ☐ STRONG
- ☐ LIMBER
- ☐ RELAXED
- ☐ ______________
- ☐ SLUGGISH
- ☐ TIRED
- ☐ WEAK
- ☐ SORE
- ☐ STRESSED
- ☐ ______________

THINGS THAT WERE FUN OR RELAXING TODAY:

____

____

____

THINGS THAT WERE HARD OR STRESSFUL TODAY:

____

____

____

OTHER THOUGHTS:

KIND THINGS I DID FOR MYSELF:

____

____

____

TIME:	AS I WOKE UP			AS I WENT TO SLEEP
MOOD:				
NOTES:				

RECORD

DATE ___/___/___

AN INTENTION FOR THE DAY:

SLEPT: FROM ___:___ TO ___:___ TOTAL HOURS: ___

☐ GOOD DREAMS ☐ BAD DREAMS ☐ NO DREAMS

NOTES:

WHAT I ATE FOR:

BREAKFAST:	LUNCH:
DINNER:	SNACKS:

NUMBER OF CUPS OF WATER I DRANK: ___

EXERCISE: ___:___ TO ___:___ TOTAL MINUTES: ___

TYPE:

OTHER ACTIVITIES:

- ☐ JOURNALING
- ☐ SOCIAL TIME
- ☐ MEDITATION
- ☐ GRATITUDE
- ☐ TIME OUTSIDE
- ☐ CREATIVE WORK
- ☐ SPIRITUAL PRACTICE
- ☐ SPA DAY
- ☐ THERAPY
- ☐ ALONE TIME
- ☐ BEING SILLY
- ☐ LEARNING SOMETHING NEW
- ☐ LISTENING TO MUSIC
- ☐ COOKING
- ☐ CLEANING
- ☐ ___________

REFLECT

PHYSICALLY, I FEEL:

- ☐ ENERGIZED
- ☐ WELL-RESTED
- ☐ STRONG
- ☐ LIMBER
- ☐ RELAXED
- ☐ ____________
- ☐ SLUGGISH
- ☐ TIRED
- ☐ WEAK
- ☐ SORE
- ☐ STRESSED
- ☐ ____________

THINGS THAT WERE FUN OR RELAXING TODAY:

____

____

____

OTHER THOUGHTS:

THINGS THAT WERE HARD OR STRESSFUL TODAY:

____

____

____

KIND THINGS I DID FOR MYSELF:

____

____

____

TIME:	AS I WOKE UP			AS I WENT TO SLEEP
MOOD:				
NOTES:				

RECORD

DATE ___/___/___

AN INTENTION FOR THE DAY:

SLEPT: FROM ___:___ TO ___:___ TOTAL HOURS:___

☐ GOOD DREAMS ☐ BAD DREAMS ☐ NO DREAMS

NOTES:

WHAT I ATE FOR:

BREAKFAST:	LUNCH:
DINNER:	SNACKS:

NUMBER OF CUPS OF WATER I DRANK: ___

EXERCISE: ___:___ TO ___:___ TOTAL MINUTES:___

TYPE:

OTHER ACTIVITIES:

- ☐ JOURNALING
- ☐ SOCIAL TIME
- ☐ MEDITATION
- ☐ GRATITUDE
- ☐ TIME OUTSIDE
- ☐ CREATIVE WORK
- ☐ SPIRITUAL PRACTICE
- ☐ SPA DAY
- ☐ THERAPY
- ☐ ALONE TIME
- ☐ BEING SILLY
- ☐ LEARNING SOMETHING NEW
- ☐ LISTENING TO MUSIC
- ☐ COOKING
- ☐ CLEANING
- ☐ ___

REFLECT

PHYSICALLY, I FEEL:

- [ ] ENERGIZED
- [ ] WELL-RESTED
- [ ] STRONG
- [ ] LIMBER
- [ ] RELAXED
- [ ] ______________
- [ ] SLUGGISH
- [ ] TIRED
- [ ] WEAK
- [ ] SORE
- [ ] STRESSED
- [ ] ______________

THINGS THAT WERE FUN OR RELAXING TODAY:

____

____

____

THINGS THAT WERE HARD OR STRESSFUL TODAY:

____

____

____

OTHER THOUGHTS:

KIND THINGS I DID FOR MYSELF:

____

____

____

TIME:	AS I WOKE UP			AS I WENT TO SLEEP
MOOD:				
NOTES:				

RECORD

DATE ___/___/___

AN INTENTION FOR THE DAY:

SLEPT: FROM ___:___ TO ___:___ TOTAL HOURS: ___

☐ GOOD DREAMS ☐ BAD DREAMS ☐ NO DREAMS

NOTES:

WHAT I ATE FOR:

BREAKFAST:	LUNCH:
DINNER:	SNACKS:

NUMBER OF CUPS OF WATER I DRANK: ___

EXERCISE: ___:___ TO ___:___ TOTAL MINUTES: ___

TYPE:

OTHER ACTIVITIES:

- ☐ JOURNALING
- ☐ SOCIAL TIME
- ☐ MEDITATION
- ☐ GRATITUDE
- ☐ TIME OUTSIDE
- ☐ CREATIVE WORK
- ☐ SPIRITUAL PRACTICE
- ☐ SPA DAY
- ☐ THERAPY
- ☐ ALONE TIME
- ☐ BEING SILLY
- ☐ LEARNING SOMETHING NEW
- ☐ LISTENING TO MUSIC
- ☐ COOKING
- ☐ CLEANING
- ☐ ___________

REFLECT

PHYSICALLY, I FEEL:

- ☐ ENERGIZED
- ☐ WELL-RESTED
- ☐ STRONG
- ☐ LIMBER
- ☐ RELAXED
- ☐ ____________
- ☐ SLUGGISH
- ☐ TIRED
- ☐ WEAK
- ☐ SORE
- ☐ STRESSED
- ☐ ____________

THINGS THAT WERE FUN OR RELAXING TODAY:

____

____

____

OTHER THOUGHTS:

THINGS THAT WERE HARD OR STRESSFUL TODAY:

____

____

____

KIND THINGS I DID FOR MYSELF:

____

____

____

TIME:	AS I WOKE UP			AS I WENT TO SLEEP
MOOD:				
NOTES:				

RECORD

DATE ___/___/___

AN INTENTION FOR THE DAY:

SLEPT: FROM ___:___ TO ___:___ TOTAL HOURS: ___

☐ GOOD DREAMS ☐ BAD DREAMS ☐ NO DREAMS

NOTES:

WHAT I ATE FOR:

BREAKFAST:	LUNCH:
DINNER:	SNACKS:

NUMBER OF CUPS OF WATER I DRANK: ___

EXERCISE: ___:___ TO ___:___ TOTAL MINUTES: ___

TYPE:

OTHER ACTIVITIES:

- ☐ JOURNALING
- ☐ SOCIAL TIME
- ☐ MEDITATION
- ☐ GRATITUDE
- ☐ TIME OUTSIDE
- ☐ CREATIVE WORK
- ☐ SPIRITUAL PRACTICE
- ☐ SPA DAY
- ☐ THERAPY
- ☐ ALONE TIME
- ☐ BEING SILLY
- ☐ LEARNING SOMETHING NEW
- ☐ LISTENING TO MUSIC
- ☐ COOKING
- ☐ CLEANING
- ☐ ___________

REFLECT

PHYSICALLY, I FEEL:

- [ ] ENERGIZED
- [ ] WELL-RESTED
- [ ] STRONG
- [ ] LIMBER
- [ ] RELAXED
- [ ] ______________
- [ ] SLUGGISH
- [ ] TIRED
- [ ] WEAK
- [ ] SORE
- [ ] STRESSED
- [ ] ______________

THINGS THAT WERE FUN OR RELAXING TODAY:

____

____

____

OTHER THOUGHTS:

THINGS THAT WERE HARD OR STRESSFUL TODAY:

____

____

____

KIND THINGS I DID FOR MYSELF:

____

____

____

TIME:	AS I WOKE UP			AS I WENT TO SLEEP
MOOD:				
NOTES:				

RECORD

DATE ___/___/___

AN INTENTION FOR THE DAY:

SLEPT: FROM ___:___ TO ___:___ TOTAL HOURS:___

☐ GOOD DREAMS ☐ BAD DREAMS ☐ NO DREAMS

NOTES:

WHAT I ATE FOR:

BREAKFAST:	LUNCH:
DINNER:	SNACKS:

NUMBER OF CUPS OF WATER I DRANK:___

EXERCISE: ___:___ TO ___:___ TOTAL MINUTES:___

TYPE:

OTHER ACTIVITIES:

☐ JOURNALING
☐ SOCIAL TIME
☐ MEDITATION
☐ GRATITUDE
☐ TIME OUTSIDE
☐ CREATIVE WORK
☐ SPIRITUAL PRACTICE
☐ SPA DAY
☐ THERAPY
☐ ALONE TIME
☐ BEING SILLY
☐ LEARNING SOMETHING NEW
☐ LISTENING TO MUSIC
☐ COOKING
☐ CLEANING
☐ ___________

REFLECT

PHYSICALLY, I FEEL:

☐ ENERGIZED	☐ SLUGGISH
☐ WELL-RESTED	☐ TIRED
☐ STRONG	☐ WEAK
☐ LIMBER	☐ SORE
☐ RELAXED	☐ STRESSED
☐ ________________	☐ ________________

THINGS THAT WERE FUN OR RELAXING TODAY:

____

____

____

OTHER THOUGHTS:

THINGS THAT WERE HARD OR STRESSFUL TODAY:

____

____

____

KIND THINGS I DID FOR MYSELF:

____

____

____

TIME:	AS I WOKE UP			AS I WENT TO SLEEP
MOOD:				
NOTES:				

RECORD

DATE ___/___/___

AN INTENTION FOR THE DAY:

SLEPT: FROM ___:___ TO ___:___ TOTAL HOURS: ___

☐ GOOD DREAMS ☐ BAD DREAMS ☐ NO DREAMS

NOTES:

WHAT I ATE FOR:

BREAKFAST:	LUNCH:
DINNER:	SNACKS:

NUMBER OF CUPS OF WATER I DRANK: ___

EXERCISE: ___:___ TO ___:___ TOTAL MINUTES: ___

TYPE:

OTHER ACTIVITIES:

☐ JOURNALING
☐ SOCIAL TIME
☐ MEDITATION
☐ GRATITUDE
☐ TIME OUTSIDE
☐ CREATIVE WORK
☐ SPIRITUAL PRACTICE
☐ SPA DAY
☐ THERAPY
☐ ALONE TIME
☐ BEING SILLY
☐ LEARNING SOMETHING NEW
☐ LISTENING TO MUSIC
☐ COOKING
☐ CLEANING
☐ ___

REFLECT

PHYSICALLY, I FEEL:

- ☐ ENERGIZED
- ☐ WELL-RESTED
- ☐ STRONG
- ☐ LIMBER
- ☐ RELAXED
- ☐ ____________
- ☐ SLUGGISH
- ☐ TIRED
- ☐ WEAK
- ☐ SORE
- ☐ STRESSED
- ☐ ____________

THINGS THAT WERE FUN OR RELAXING TODAY:

____

____

____

THINGS THAT WERE HARD OR STRESSFUL TODAY:

____

____

____

OTHER THOUGHTS:

KIND THINGS I DID FOR MYSELF:

____

____

____

TIME:	AS I WOKE UP			AS I WENT TO SLEEP
MOOD:				
NOTES:				

RECORD

DATE ___/___/___

AN INTENTION FOR THE DAY:

SLEPT: FROM ___:___ TO ___:___ TOTAL HOURS: ___

☐ GOOD DREAMS ☐ BAD DREAMS ☐ NO DREAMS

NOTES:

WHAT I ATE FOR:

BREAKFAST:	LUNCH:
DINNER:	SNACKS:

NUMBER OF CUPS OF WATER I DRANK: ___

EXERCISE: ___:___ TO ___:___ TOTAL MINUTES: ___

TYPE:

OTHER ACTIVITIES:

☐ JOURNALING	☐ SPIRITUAL PRACTICE	☐ LEARNING SOMETHING NEW
☐ SOCIAL TIME	☐ SPA DAY	☐ LISTENING TO MUSIC
☐ MEDITATION	☐ THERAPY	☐ COOKING
☐ GRATITUDE	☐ ALONE TIME	☐ CLEANING
☐ TIME OUTSIDE	☐ BEING SILLY	☐ ___________
☐ CREATIVE WORK		

REFLECT

PHYSICALLY, I FEEL:

- ☐ ENERGIZED
- ☐ WELL-RESTED
- ☐ STRONG
- ☐ LIMBER
- ☐ RELAXED
- ☐ ______________
- ☐ SLUGGISH
- ☐ TIRED
- ☐ WEAK
- ☐ SORE
- ☐ STRESSED
- ☐ ______________

THINGS THAT WERE FUN OR RELAXING TODAY:

____

____

____

THINGS THAT WERE HARD OR STRESSFUL TODAY:

____

____

____

OTHER THOUGHTS:

KIND THINGS I DID FOR MYSELF:

____

____

____

TIME:	AS I WOKE UP			AS I WENT TO SLEEP
MOOD:				
NOTES:				

RECORD

DATE ___/___/___

AN INTENTION FOR THE DAY:

SLEPT: FROM ___:___ TO ___:___ TOTAL HOURS:___

☐ GOOD DREAMS ☐ BAD DREAMS ☐ NO DREAMS

NOTES:

WHAT I ATE FOR:

BREAKFAST:	LUNCH:
DINNER:	SNACKS:

NUMBER OF CUPS OF WATER I DRANK:___

EXERCISE: ___:___ TO ___:___ TOTAL MINUTES:___

TYPE:

OTHER ACTIVITIES:

- ☐ JOURNALING
- ☐ SOCIAL TIME
- ☐ MEDITATION
- ☐ GRATITUDE
- ☐ TIME OUTSIDE
- ☐ CREATIVE WORK
- ☐ SPIRITUAL PRACTICE
- ☐ SPA DAY
- ☐ THERAPY
- ☐ ALONE TIME
- ☐ BEING SILLY
- ☐ LEARNING SOMETHING NEW
- ☐ LISTENING TO MUSIC
- ☐ COOKING
- ☐ CLEANING
- ☐ ___________

REFLECT

PHYSICALLY, I FEEL:

☐ ENERGIZED	☐ SLUGGISH
☐ WELL-RESTED	☐ TIRED
☐ STRONG	☐ WEAK
☐ LIMBER	☐ SORE
☐ RELAXED	☐ STRESSED
☐ ____________	☐ ____________

THINGS THAT WERE FUN OR RELAXING TODAY:

OTHER THOUGHTS:

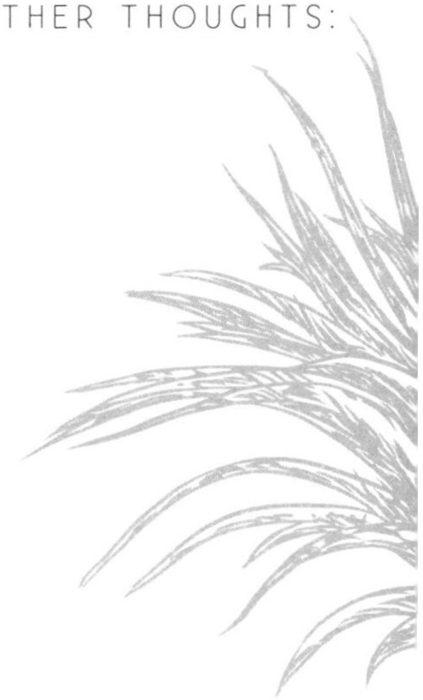

THINGS THAT WERE HARD OR STRESSFUL TODAY:

KIND THINGS I DID FOR MYSELF:

TIME:	AS I WOKE UP			AS I WENT TO SLEEP
MOOD:				
NOTES:				

RECORD

DATE ___/___/___

AN INTENTION FOR THE DAY:

SLEPT: FROM ___:___ TO ___:___ TOTAL HOURS:___

☐ GOOD DREAMS ☐ BAD DREAMS ☐ NO DREAMS

NOTES:

WHAT I ATE FOR:

BREAKFAST:	LUNCH:
DINNER:	SNACKS:

NUMBER OF CUPS OF WATER I DRANK:___

EXERCISE: ___:___ TO ___:___ TOTAL MINUTES:___

TYPE:

OTHER ACTIVITIES:

- ☐ JOURNALING
- ☐ SOCIAL TIME
- ☐ MEDITATION
- ☐ GRATITUDE
- ☐ TIME OUTSIDE
- ☐ CREATIVE WORK
- ☐ SPIRITUAL PRACTICE
- ☐ SPA DAY
- ☐ THERAPY
- ☐ ALONE TIME
- ☐ BEING SILLY
- ☐ LEARNING SOMETHING NEW
- ☐ LISTENING TO MUSIC
- ☐ COOKING
- ☐ CLEANING
- ☐ ___________

REFLECT

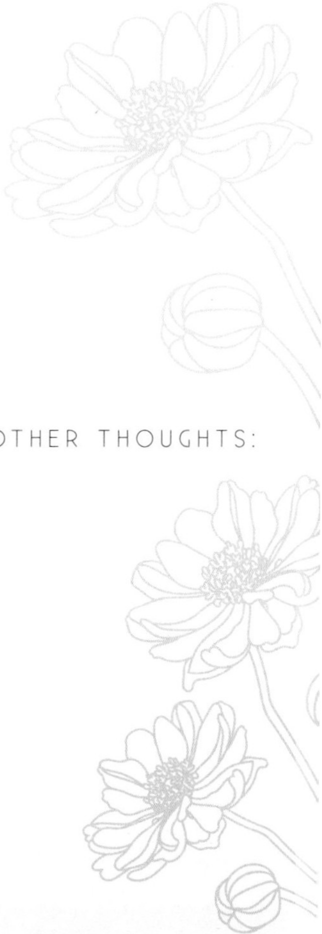

PHYSICALLY, I FEEL:

- [ ] ENERGIZED
- [ ] WELL-RESTED
- [ ] STRONG
- [ ] LIMBER
- [ ] RELAXED
- [ ] ______________
- [ ] SLUGGISH
- [ ] TIRED
- [ ] WEAK
- [ ] SORE
- [ ] STRESSED
- [ ] ______________

THINGS THAT WERE FUN OR RELAXING TODAY:

____

____

____

OTHER THOUGHTS:

THINGS THAT WERE HARD OR STRESSFUL TODAY:

____

____

____

KIND THINGS I DID FOR MYSELF:

____

____

____

TIME:	AS I WOKE UP			AS I WENT TO SLEEP
MOOD:				
NOTES:				

RECORD

DATE ___/___/___

AN INTENTION FOR THE DAY:

SLEPT: FROM ___:___ TO ___:___ TOTAL HOURS:___

☐ GOOD DREAMS ☐ BAD DREAMS ☐ NO DREAMS

NOTES:

WHAT I ATE FOR:

BREAKFAST:	LUNCH:
DINNER:	SNACKS:

NUMBER OF CUPS OF WATER I DRANK:___

EXERCISE: ___:___ TO ___:___ TOTAL MINUTES:___

TYPE:

OTHER ACTIVITIES:

- ☐ JOURNALING
- ☐ SOCIAL TIME
- ☐ MEDITATION
- ☐ GRATITUDE
- ☐ TIME OUTSIDE
- ☐ CREATIVE WORK
- ☐ SPIRITUAL PRACTICE
- ☐ SPA DAY
- ☐ THERAPY
- ☐ ALONE TIME
- ☐ BEING SILLY
- ☐ LEARNING SOMETHING NEW
- ☐ LISTENING TO MUSIC
- ☐ COOKING
- ☐ CLEANING
- ☐ ___________

REFLECT

PHYSICALLY, I FEEL:

- [ ] ENERGIZED
- [ ] WELL-RESTED
- [ ] STRONG
- [ ] LIMBER
- [ ] RELAXED
- [ ] ____________
- [ ] SLUGGISH
- [ ] TIRED
- [ ] WEAK
- [ ] SORE
- [ ] STRESSED
- [ ] ____________

THINGS THAT WERE FUN OR RELAXING TODAY:

____

____

____

OTHER THOUGHTS:

THINGS THAT WERE HARD OR STRESSFUL TODAY:

____

____

____

KIND THINGS I DID FOR MYSELF:

____

____

____

TIME:	AS I WOKE UP			AS I WENT TO SLEEP
MOOD:				
NOTES:				

RECORD

DATE ___/___/___

AN INTENTION FOR THE DAY:

SLEPT: FROM ___:___ TO ___:___ TOTAL HOURS: ___

☐ GOOD DREAMS ☐ BAD DREAMS ☐ NO DREAMS

NOTES:

WHAT I ATE FOR:

BREAKFAST:	LUNCH:
DINNER:	SNACKS:

NUMBER OF CUPS OF WATER I DRANK: ___

EXERCISE: ___:___ TO ___:___ TOTAL MINUTES: ___

TYPE:

OTHER ACTIVITIES:

- ☐ JOURNALING
- ☐ SOCIAL TIME
- ☐ MEDITATION
- ☐ GRATITUDE
- ☐ TIME OUTSIDE
- ☐ CREATIVE WORK
- ☐ SPIRITUAL PRACTICE
- ☐ SPA DAY
- ☐ THERAPY
- ☐ ALONE TIME
- ☐ BEING SILLY
- ☐ LEARNING SOMETHING NEW
- ☐ LISTENING TO MUSIC
- ☐ COOKING
- ☐ CLEANING
- ☐ ___________

REFLECT

PHYSICALLY, I FEEL:

- [ ] ENERGIZED
- [ ] WELL-RESTED
- [ ] STRONG
- [ ] LIMBER
- [ ] RELAXED
- [ ] ____________
- [ ] SLUGGISH
- [ ] TIRED
- [ ] WEAK
- [ ] SORE
- [ ] STRESSED
- [ ] ____________

THINGS THAT WERE FUN OR RELAXING TODAY:

____

____

____

OTHER THOUGHTS:

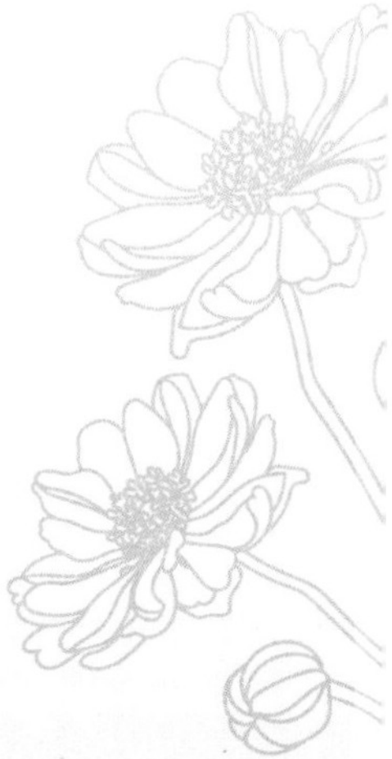

THINGS THAT WERE HARD OR STRESSFUL TODAY:

____

____

____

KIND THINGS I DID FOR MYSELF:

____

____

____

TIME:	AS I WOKE UP			AS I WENT TO SLEEP
MOOD:				
NOTES:				

RECORD

DATE ___/___/___

AN INTENTION FOR THE DAY:

SLEPT: FROM ___:___ TO ___:___ TOTAL HOURS:___

☐ GOOD DREAMS ☐ BAD DREAMS ☐ NO DREAMS

NOTES:

WHAT I ATE FOR:

BREAKFAST:	LUNCH:
DINNER:	SNACKS:

NUMBER OF CUPS OF WATER I DRANK:___

EXERCISE: ___:___ TO ___:___ TOTAL MINUTES:___
TYPE:

OTHER ACTIVITIES:

- ☐ JOURNALING
- ☐ SOCIAL TIME
- ☐ MEDITATION
- ☐ GRATITUDE
- ☐ TIME OUTSIDE
- ☐ CREATIVE WORK
- ☐ SPIRITUAL PRACTICE
- ☐ SPA DAY
- ☐ THERAPY
- ☐ ALONE TIME
- ☐ BEING SILLY
- ☐ LEARNING SOMETHING NEW
- ☐ LISTENING TO MUSIC
- ☐ COOKING
- ☐ CLEANING
- ☐ ___________

REFLECT

PHYSICALLY, I FEEL:

- ☐ ENERGIZED
- ☐ WELL-RESTED
- ☐ STRONG
- ☐ LIMBER
- ☐ RELAXED
- ☐ ______________
- ☐ SLUGGISH
- ☐ TIRED
- ☐ WEAK
- ☐ SORE
- ☐ STRESSED
- ☐ ______________

THINGS THAT WERE FUN OR RELAXING TODAY:

____

____

____

OTHER THOUGHTS:

THINGS THAT WERE HARD OR STRESSFUL TODAY:

____

____

____

KIND THINGS I DID FOR MYSELF:

____

____

____

TIME:	AS I WOKE UP			AS I WENT TO SLEEP
MOOD:				
NOTES:				

RECORD

DATE ___/___/___

AN INTENTION FOR THE DAY:

SLEPT: FROM ___:___ TO ___:___ TOTAL HOURS:___

☐ GOOD DREAMS ☐ BAD DREAMS ☐ NO DREAMS

NOTES:

WHAT I ATE FOR:

BREAKFAST:	LUNCH:
DINNER:	SNACKS:

NUMBER OF CUPS OF WATER I DRANK:___

EXERCISE: ___:___ TO ___:___ TOTAL MINUTES:___

TYPE:

OTHER ACTIVITIES:

- ☐ JOURNALING
- ☐ SOCIAL TIME
- ☐ MEDITATION
- ☐ GRATITUDE
- ☐ TIME OUTSIDE
- ☐ CREATIVE WORK
- ☐ SPIRITUAL PRACTICE
- ☐ SPA DAY
- ☐ THERAPY
- ☐ ALONE TIME
- ☐ BEING SILLY
- ☐ LEARNING SOMETHING NEW
- ☐ LISTENING TO MUSIC
- ☐ COOKING
- ☐ CLEANING
- ☐ ________

REFLECT

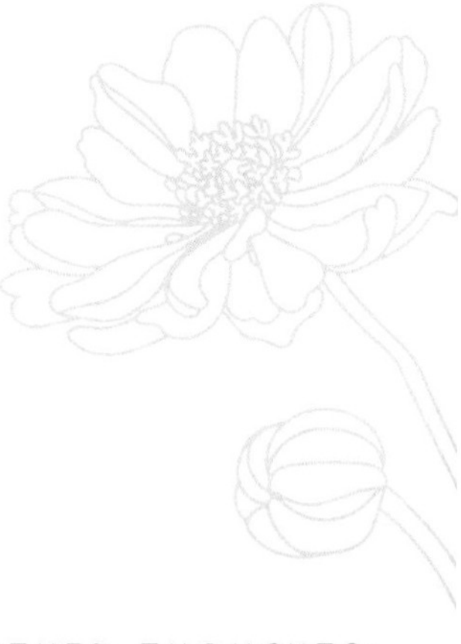

PHYSICALLY, I FEEL:

- ☐ ENERGIZED
- ☐ WELL-RESTED
- ☐ STRONG
- ☐ LIMBER
- ☐ RELAXED
- ☐ ____________
- ☐ SLUGGISH
- ☐ TIRED
- ☐ WEAK
- ☐ SORE
- ☐ STRESSED
- ☐ ____________

THINGS THAT WERE FUN OR RELAXING TODAY:

____

____

____

THINGS THAT WERE HARD OR STRESSFUL TODAY:

____

____

____

OTHER THOUGHTS:

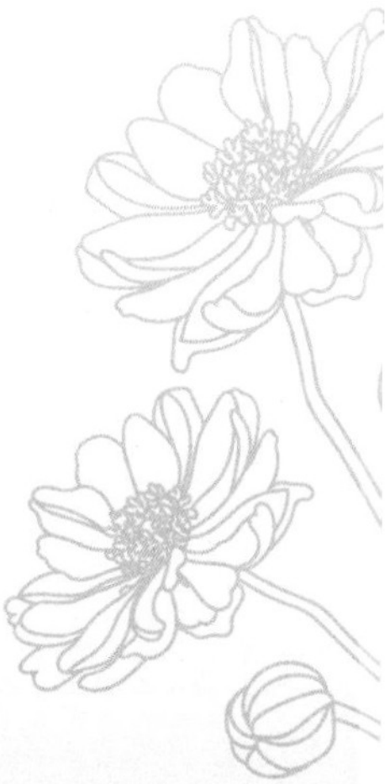

KIND THINGS I DID FOR MYSELF:

____

____

____

TIME:	AS I WOKE UP			AS I WENT TO SLEEP
MOOD:				
NOTES:				

RECORD

DATE ___/___/___

AN INTENTION FOR THE DAY:

SLEPT: FROM ___:___ TO ___:___ TOTAL HOURS:___

☐ GOOD DREAMS ☐ BAD DREAMS ☐ NO DREAMS

NOTES:

WHAT I ATE FOR:

BREAKFAST:	LUNCH:
DINNER:	SNACKS:

NUMBER OF CUPS OF WATER I DRANK:___

EXERCISE: ___:___ TO ___:___ TOTAL MINUTES:___

TYPE:

OTHER ACTIVITIES:

☐ JOURNALING
☐ SOCIAL TIME
☐ MEDITATION
☐ GRATITUDE
☐ TIME OUTSIDE
☐ CREATIVE WORK
☐ SPIRITUAL PRACTICE
☐ SPA DAY
☐ THERAPY
☐ ALONE TIME
☐ BEING SILLY
☐ LEARNING SOMETHING NEW
☐ LISTENING TO MUSIC
☐ COOKING
☐ CLEANING
☐ ____________

REFLECT

PHYSICALLY, I FEEL:

☐ ENERGIZED	☐ SLUGGISH
☐ WELL-RESTED	☐ TIRED
☐ STRONG	☐ WEAK
☐ LIMBER	☐ SORE
☐ RELAXED	☐ STRESSED
☐ ______________	☐ ______________

THINGS THAT WERE FUN OR RELAXING TODAY:

OTHER THOUGHTS:

THINGS THAT WERE HARD OR STRESSFUL TODAY:

KIND THINGS I DID FOR MYSELF:

TIME:	AS I WOKE UP			AS I WENT TO SLEEP
MOOD:				
NOTES:				

RECORD

DATE ___/___/___

AN INTENTION FOR THE DAY:

SLEPT: FROM ___:___ TO ___:___ TOTAL HOURS:___

☐ GOOD DREAMS ☐ BAD DREAMS ☐ NO DREAMS

NOTES:

WHAT I ATE FOR:

BREAKFAST:	LUNCH:
DINNER:	SNACKS:

NUMBER OF CUPS OF WATER I DRANK:___

EXERCISE: ___:___ TO ___:___ TOTAL MINUTES:___

TYPE:

OTHER ACTIVITIES:

- ☐ JOURNALING
- ☐ SOCIAL TIME
- ☐ MEDITATION
- ☐ GRATITUDE
- ☐ TIME OUTSIDE
- ☐ CREATIVE WORK
- ☐ SPIRITUAL PRACTICE
- ☐ SPA DAY
- ☐ THERAPY
- ☐ ALONE TIME
- ☐ BEING SILLY
- ☐ LEARNING SOMETHING NEW
- ☐ LISTENING TO MUSIC
- ☐ COOKING
- ☐ CLEANING
- ☐ ___________

REFLECT

PHYSICALLY, I FEEL:

- ☐ ENERGIZED
- ☐ WELL-RESTED
- ☐ STRONG
- ☐ LIMBER
- ☐ RELAXED
- ☐ ____________
- ☐ SLUGGISH
- ☐ TIRED
- ☐ WEAK
- ☐ SORE
- ☐ STRESSED
- ☐ ____________

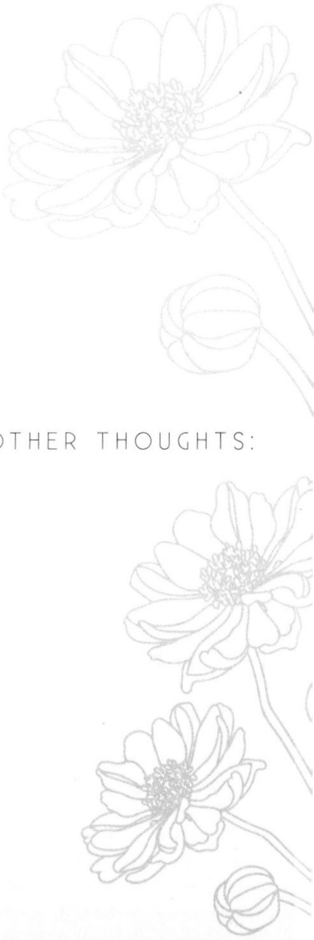

THINGS THAT WERE FUN OR RELAXING TODAY:

OTHER THOUGHTS:

THINGS THAT WERE HARD OR STRESSFUL TODAY:

KIND THINGS I DID FOR MYSELF:

TIME:	AS I WOKE UP			AS I WENT TO SLEEP
MOOD:				
NOTES:				

RECORD

DATE ___/___/___

AN INTENTION FOR THE DAY:

SLEPT: FROM ___:___ TO ___:___ TOTAL HOURS: ___

☐ GOOD DREAMS ☐ BAD DREAMS ☐ NO DREAMS

NOTES:

WHAT I ATE FOR:

BREAKFAST:	LUNCH:
DINNER:	SNACKS:

NUMBER OF CUPS OF WATER I DRANK: ___

EXERCISE: ___:___ TO ___:___ TOTAL MINUTES: ___

TYPE:

OTHER ACTIVITIES:

☐ JOURNALING
☐ SOCIAL TIME
☐ MEDITATION
☐ GRATITUDE
☐ TIME OUTSIDE
☐ CREATIVE WORK
☐ SPIRITUAL PRACTICE
☐ SPA DAY
☐ THERAPY
☐ ALONE TIME
☐ BEING SILLY
☐ LEARNING SOMETHING NEW
☐ LISTENING TO MUSIC
☐ COOKING
☐ CLEANING
☐ ___________

REFLECT

PHYSICALLY, I FEEL:

- [ ] ENERGIZED
- [ ] WELL-RESTED
- [ ] STRONG
- [ ] LIMBER
- [ ] RELAXED
- [ ] ____________
- [ ] SLUGGISH
- [ ] TIRED
- [ ] WEAK
- [ ] SORE
- [ ] STRESSED
- [ ] ____________

THINGS THAT WERE FUN OR RELAXING TODAY:

____

____

____

THINGS THAT WERE HARD OR STRESSFUL TODAY:

____

____

____

OTHER THOUGHTS:

KIND THINGS I DID FOR MYSELF:

____

____

____

TIME:	AS I WOKE UP			AS I WENT TO SLEEP
MOOD:				
NOTES:				

RECORD

DATE ___/___/___

AN INTENTION FOR THE DAY:

SLEPT: FROM ___:___ TO ___:___ TOTAL HOURS:___

☐ GOOD DREAMS ☐ BAD DREAMS ☐ NO DREAMS

NOTES:

WHAT I ATE FOR:

BREAKFAST:	LUNCH:
DINNER:	SNACKS:

NUMBER OF CUPS OF WATER I DRANK:___

EXERCISE: ___:___ TO ___:___ TOTAL MINUTES:___

TYPE:

OTHER ACTIVITIES:

- ☐ JOURNALING
- ☐ SOCIAL TIME
- ☐ MEDITATION
- ☐ GRATITUDE
- ☐ TIME OUTSIDE
- ☐ CREATIVE WORK
- ☐ SPIRITUAL PRACTICE
- ☐ SPA DAY
- ☐ THERAPY
- ☐ ALONE TIME
- ☐ BEING SILLY
- ☐ LEARNING SOMETHING NEW
- ☐ LISTENING TO MUSIC
- ☐ COOKING
- ☐ CLEANING
- ☐ ___________

REFLECT

PHYSICALLY, I FEEL:

☐ ENERGIZED	☐ SLUGGISH
☐ WELL-RESTED	☐ TIRED
☐ STRONG	☐ WEAK
☐ LIMBER	☐ SORE
☐ RELAXED	☐ STRESSED
☐ ____________	☐ ____________

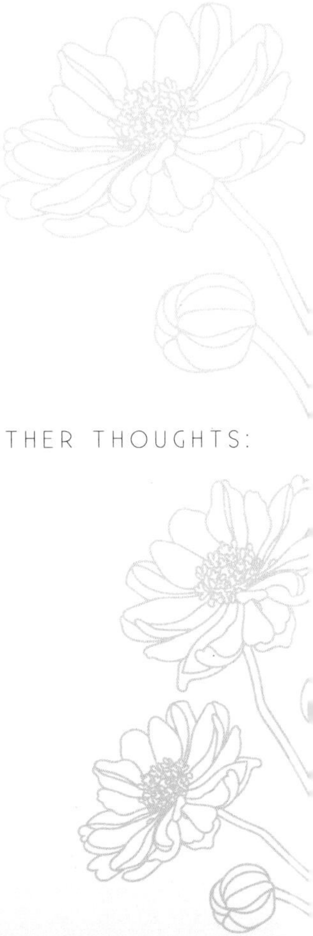

THINGS THAT WERE FUN OR RELAXING TODAY:

OTHER THOUGHTS:

THINGS THAT WERE HARD OR STRESSFUL TODAY:

KIND THINGS I DID FOR MYSELF:

TIME:	AS I WOKE UP			AS I WENT TO SLEEP
MOOD:				
NOTES:				

RECORD

DATE ___/___/___

AN INTENTION FOR THE DAY:

SLEPT: FROM ___:___ TO ___:___ TOTAL HOURS:___

☐ GOOD DREAMS ☐ BAD DREAMS ☐ NO DREAMS

NOTES:

WHAT I ATE FOR:

BREAKFAST:	LUNCH:
DINNER:	SNACKS:

NUMBER OF CUPS OF WATER I DRANK:___

EXERCISE: ___:___ TO ___:___ TOTAL MINUTES:___

TYPE:

OTHER ACTIVITIES:

- ☐ JOURNALING
- ☐ SOCIAL TIME
- ☐ MEDITATION
- ☐ GRATITUDE
- ☐ TIME OUTSIDE
- ☐ CREATIVE WORK
- ☐ SPIRITUAL PRACTICE
- ☐ SPA DAY
- ☐ THERAPY
- ☐ ALONE TIME
- ☐ BEING SILLY
- ☐ LEARNING SOMETHING NEW
- ☐ LISTENING TO MUSIC
- ☐ COOKING
- ☐ CLEANING
- ☐ ___________

REFLECT

PHYSICALLY, I FEEL:

☐ ENERGIZED	☐ SLUGGISH
☐ WELL-RESTED	☐ TIRED
☐ STRONG	☐ WEAK
☐ LIMBER	☐ SORE
☐ RELAXED	☐ STRESSED
☐ ____________	☐ ____________

THINGS THAT WERE FUN OR RELAXING TODAY:

____

____

____

THINGS THAT WERE HARD OR STRESSFUL TODAY:

____

____

____

OTHER THOUGHTS:

KIND THINGS I DID FOR MYSELF:

____

____

____

TIME:	AS I WOKE UP			AS I WENT TO SLEEP
MOOD:				
NOTES:				

RECORD

DATE ___/___/___

AN INTENTION FOR THE DAY:

SLEPT: FROM ___:___ TO ___:___ TOTAL HOURS: ___

☐ GOOD DREAMS ☐ BAD DREAMS ☐ NO DREAMS

NOTES:

WHAT I ATE FOR:

BREAKFAST:	LUNCH:
DINNER:	SNACKS:

NUMBER OF CUPS OF WATER I DRANK: ___

EXERCISE: ___:___ TO ___:___ TOTAL MINUTES: ___

TYPE:

OTHER ACTIVITIES:

☐ JOURNALING
☐ SOCIAL TIME
☐ MEDITATION
☐ GRATITUDE
☐ TIME OUTSIDE
☐ CREATIVE WORK
☐ SPIRITUAL PRACTICE
☐ SPA DAY
☐ THERAPY
☐ ALONE TIME
☐ BEING SILLY
☐ LEARNING SOMETHING NEW
☐ LISTENING TO MUSIC
☐ COOKING
☐ CLEANING
☐ ___

REFLECT

PHYSICALLY, I FEEL:

- ☐ ENERGIZED
- ☐ WELL-RESTED
- ☐ STRONG
- ☐ LIMBER
- ☐ RELAXED
- ☐ ____________
- ☐ SLUGGISH
- ☐ TIRED
- ☐ WEAK
- ☐ SORE
- ☐ STRESSED
- ☐ ____________

THINGS THAT WERE FUN OR RELAXING TODAY:

____

____

____

THINGS THAT WERE HARD OR STRESSFUL TODAY:

____

____

____

OTHER THOUGHTS:

KIND THINGS I DID FOR MYSELF:

____

____

____

TIME:	AS I WOKE UP			AS I WENT TO SLEEP
MOOD:				
NOTES:				

RECORD

DATE ___/___/___

AN INTENTION FOR THE DAY:

SLEPT: FROM ___:___ TO ___:___ TOTAL HOURS: ___

☐ GOOD DREAMS ☐ BAD DREAMS ☐ NO DREAMS

NOTES:

WHAT I ATE FOR:

BREAKFAST:	LUNCH:
DINNER:	SNACKS:

NUMBER OF CUPS OF WATER I DRANK: ___

EXERCISE: ___:___ TO ___:___ TOTAL MINUTES: ___

TYPE:

OTHER ACTIVITIES:

- ☐ JOURNALING
- ☐ SOCIAL TIME
- ☐ MEDITATION
- ☐ GRATITUDE
- ☐ TIME OUTSIDE
- ☐ CREATIVE WORK
- ☐ SPIRITUAL PRACTICE
- ☐ SPA DAY
- ☐ THERAPY
- ☐ ALONE TIME
- ☐ BEING SILLY
- ☐ LEARNING SOMETHING NEW
- ☐ LISTENING TO MUSIC
- ☐ COOKING
- ☐ CLEANING
- ☐ ________

REFLECT

PHYSICALLY, I FEEL:

- [ ] ENERGIZED
- [ ] WELL-RESTED
- [ ] STRONG
- [ ] LIMBER
- [ ] RELAXED
- [ ] ______________
- [ ] SLUGGISH
- [ ] TIRED
- [ ] WEAK
- [ ] SORE
- [ ] STRESSED
- [ ] ______________

THINGS THAT WERE FUN OR RELAXING TODAY:

____

____

____

THINGS THAT WERE HARD OR STRESSFUL TODAY:

____

____

____

OTHER THOUGHTS:

KIND THINGS I DID FOR MYSELF:

____

____

____

TIME:	AS I WOKE UP			AS I WENT TO SLEEP
MOOD:				
NOTES:				

RECORD

DATE ___/___/___

AN INTENTION FOR THE DAY:

SLEPT: FROM ___:___ TO ___:___ TOTAL HOURS: ___

☐ GOOD DREAMS ☐ BAD DREAMS ☐ NO DREAMS

NOTES:

WHAT I ATE FOR:

BREAKFAST:	LUNCH:
DINNER:	SNACKS:

NUMBER OF CUPS OF WATER I DRANK: ___

EXERCISE: ___:___ TO ___:___ TOTAL MINUTES: ___

TYPE:

OTHER ACTIVITIES:

- ☐ JOURNALING
- ☐ SOCIAL TIME
- ☐ MEDITATION
- ☐ GRATITUDE
- ☐ TIME OUTSIDE
- ☐ CREATIVE WORK
- ☐ SPIRITUAL PRACTICE
- ☐ SPA DAY
- ☐ THERAPY
- ☐ ALONE TIME
- ☐ BEING SILLY
- ☐ LEARNING SOMETHING NEW
- ☐ LISTENING TO MUSIC
- ☐ COOKING
- ☐ CLEANING
- ☐ ___

REFLECT

PHYSICALLY, I FEEL:

- [ ] ENERGIZED
- [ ] WELL-RESTED
- [ ] STRONG
- [ ] LIMBER
- [ ] RELAXED
- [ ] ______________
- [ ] SLUGGISH
- [ ] TIRED
- [ ] WEAK
- [ ] SORE
- [ ] STRESSED
- [ ] ______________

THINGS THAT WERE FUN OR RELAXING TODAY:

____

____

____

THINGS THAT WERE HARD OR STRESSFUL TODAY:

____

____

____

OTHER THOUGHTS:

KIND THINGS I DID FOR MYSELF:

____

____

____

TIME:	AS I WOKE UP			AS I WENT TO SLEEP
MOOD:				
NOTES:				

RECORD

DATE ___/___/___

AN INTENTION FOR THE DAY:

SLEPT: FROM ___:___ TO ___:___ TOTAL HOURS: ___

☐ GOOD DREAMS ☐ BAD DREAMS ☐ NO DREAMS

NOTES:

WHAT I ATE FOR:

BREAKFAST:	LUNCH:
DINNER:	SNACKS:

NUMBER OF CUPS OF WATER I DRANK: ___

EXERCISE: ___:___ TO ___:___ TOTAL MINUTES: ___

TYPE:

OTHER ACTIVITIES:

- ☐ JOURNALING
- ☐ SOCIAL TIME
- ☐ MEDITATION
- ☐ GRATITUDE
- ☐ TIME OUTSIDE
- ☐ CREATIVE WORK
- ☐ SPIRITUAL PRACTICE
- ☐ SPA DAY
- ☐ THERAPY
- ☐ ALONE TIME
- ☐ BEING SILLY
- ☐ LEARNING SOMETHING NEW
- ☐ LISTENING TO MUSIC
- ☐ COOKING
- ☐ CLEANING
- ☐ __________

REFLECT

PHYSICALLY, I FEEL:

☐ ENERGIZED	☐ SLUGGISH
☐ WELL-RESTED	☐ TIRED
☐ STRONG	☐ WEAK
☐ LIMBER	☐ SORE
☐ RELAXED	☐ STRESSED
☐ ______________	☐ ______________

THINGS THAT WERE FUN OR RELAXING TODAY:

____

____

____

OTHER THOUGHTS:

THINGS THAT WERE HARD OR STRESSFUL TODAY:

____

____

____

KIND THINGS I DID FOR MYSELF:

____

____

____

TIME:	AS I WOKE UP			AS I WENT TO SLEEP
MOOD:				
NOTES:				

RECORD

DATE ___/___/___

AN INTENTION FOR THE DAY:

SLEPT: FROM ___:___ TO ___:___ TOTAL HOURS: ___

☐ GOOD DREAMS ☐ BAD DREAMS ☐ NO DREAMS

NOTES:

WHAT I ATE FOR:

BREAKFAST:	LUNCH:
DINNER:	SNACKS:

NUMBER OF CUPS OF WATER I DRANK: ___

EXERCISE: ___:___ TO ___:___ TOTAL MINUTES: ___

TYPE:

OTHER ACTIVITIES:

- ☐ JOURNALING
- ☐ SOCIAL TIME
- ☐ MEDITATION
- ☐ GRATITUDE
- ☐ TIME OUTSIDE
- ☐ CREATIVE WORK
- ☐ SPIRITUAL PRACTICE
- ☐ SPA DAY
- ☐ THERAPY
- ☐ ALONE TIME
- ☐ BEING SILLY
- ☐ LEARNING SOMETHING NEW
- ☐ LISTENING TO MUSIC
- ☐ COOKING
- ☐ CLEANING
- ☐ __________

REFLECT

PHYSICALLY, I FEEL:

- ☐ ENERGIZED
- ☐ WELL-RESTED
- ☐ STRONG
- ☐ LIMBER
- ☐ RELAXED
- ☐ ________
- ☐ SLUGGISH
- ☐ TIRED
- ☐ WEAK
- ☐ SORE
- ☐ STRESSED
- ☐ ________

THINGS THAT WERE FUN OR RELAXING TODAY:

____

____

____

THINGS THAT WERE HARD OR STRESSFUL TODAY:

____

____

____

OTHER THOUGHTS:

KIND THINGS I DID FOR MYSELF:

____

____

____

TIME:	AS I WOKE UP			AS I WENT TO SLEEP
MOOD:				
NOTES:				

RECORD

DATE ___/___/___

AN INTENTION FOR THE DAY:

SLEPT: FROM ___:___ TO ___:___ TOTAL HOURS: ___

☐ GOOD DREAMS ☐ BAD DREAMS ☐ NO DREAMS

NOTES:

WHAT I ATE FOR:

BREAKFAST:	LUNCH:
DINNER:	SNACKS:

NUMBER OF CUPS OF WATER I DRANK: ___

EXERCISE: ___:___ TO ___:___ TOTAL MINUTES: ___

TYPE:

OTHER ACTIVITIES:

- ☐ JOURNALING
- ☐ SOCIAL TIME
- ☐ MEDITATION
- ☐ GRATITUDE
- ☐ TIME OUTSIDE
- ☐ CREATIVE WORK
- ☐ SPIRITUAL PRACTICE
- ☐ SPA DAY
- ☐ THERAPY
- ☐ ALONE TIME
- ☐ BEING SILLY
- ☐ LEARNING SOMETHING NEW
- ☐ LISTENING TO MUSIC
- ☐ COOKING
- ☐ CLEANING
- ☐ __________

REFLECT

PHYSICALLY, I FEEL:

- [ ] ENERGIZED
- [ ] WELL-RESTED
- [ ] STRONG
- [ ] LIMBER
- [ ] RELAXED
- [ ] ______________
- [ ] SLUGGISH
- [ ] TIRED
- [ ] WEAK
- [ ] SORE
- [ ] STRESSED
- [ ] ______________

THINGS THAT WERE FUN OR RELAXING TODAY:

____

____

____

THINGS THAT WERE HARD OR STRESSFUL TODAY:

____

____

____

OTHER THOUGHTS:

KIND THINGS I DID FOR MYSELF:

____

____

____

TIME:	AS I WOKE UP			AS I WENT TO SLEEP
MOOD:				
NOTES:				

RECORD

DATE ___/___/___

AN INTENTION FOR THE DAY:

SLEPT: FROM ___:___ TO ___:___ TOTAL HOURS:___

☐ GOOD DREAMS ☐ BAD DREAMS ☐ NO DREAMS

NOTES:

WHAT I ATE FOR:

BREAKFAST:	LUNCH:
DINNER:	SNACKS:

NUMBER OF CUPS OF WATER I DRANK:___

EXERCISE: ___:___ TO ___:___ TOTAL MINUTES:___

TYPE:

OTHER ACTIVITIES:

☐ JOURNALING
☐ SOCIAL TIME
☐ MEDITATION
☐ GRATITUDE
☐ TIME OUTSIDE
☐ CREATIVE WORK
☐ SPIRITUAL PRACTICE
☐ SPA DAY
☐ THERAPY
☐ ALONE TIME
☐ BEING SILLY
☐ LEARNING SOMETHING NEW
☐ LISTENING TO MUSIC
☐ COOKING
☐ CLEANING
☐ ___________

REFLECT

PHYSICALLY, I FEEL:

- [ ] ENERGIZED
- [ ] WELL-RESTED
- [ ] STRONG
- [ ] LIMBER
- [ ] RELAXED
- [ ] ______
- [ ] SLUGGISH
- [ ] TIRED
- [ ] WEAK
- [ ] SORE
- [ ] STRESSED
- [ ] ______

THINGS THAT WERE FUN OR RELAXING TODAY:

______

______

______

THINGS THAT WERE HARD OR STRESSFUL TODAY:

______

______

______

OTHER THOUGHTS:

KIND THINGS I DID FOR MYSELF:

______

______

______

TIME:	AS I WOKE UP			AS I WENT TO SLEEP
MOOD:				
NOTES:				

RECORD

DATE ___/___/___

AN INTENTION FOR THE DAY:

SLEPT: FROM ___:___ TO ___:___ TOTAL HOURS:___

☐ GOOD DREAMS ☐ BAD DREAMS ☐ NO DREAMS

NOTES:

WHAT I ATE FOR:

BREAKFAST:	LUNCH:
DINNER:	SNACKS:

NUMBER OF CUPS OF WATER I DRANK:___

EXERCISE: ___:___ TO ___:___ TOTAL MINUTES:___

TYPE:

OTHER ACTIVITIES:

- ☐ JOURNALING
- ☐ SOCIAL TIME
- ☐ MEDITATION
- ☐ GRATITUDE
- ☐ TIME OUTSIDE
- ☐ CREATIVE WORK
- ☐ SPIRITUAL PRACTICE
- ☐ SPA DAY
- ☐ THERAPY
- ☐ ALONE TIME
- ☐ BEING SILLY
- ☐ LEARNING SOMETHING NEW
- ☐ LISTENING TO MUSIC
- ☐ COOKING
- ☐ CLEANING
- ☐ ___________

REFLECT

PHYSICALLY, I FEEL:

- [ ] ENERGIZED
- [ ] WELL-RESTED
- [ ] STRONG
- [ ] LIMBER
- [ ] RELAXED
- [ ] ____________
- [ ] SLUGGISH
- [ ] TIRED
- [ ] WEAK
- [ ] SORE
- [ ] STRESSED
- [ ] ____________

THINGS THAT WERE FUN OR RELAXING TODAY:

____

____

____

THINGS THAT WERE HARD OR STRESSFUL TODAY:

____

____

____

OTHER THOUGHTS:

KIND THINGS I DID FOR MYSELF:

____

____

____

TIME:	AS I WOKE UP			AS I WENT TO SLEEP
MOOD:				
NOTES:				

RECORD

DATE ___/___/___

AN INTENTION FOR THE DAY:

SLEPT: FROM ___:___ TO ___:___ TOTAL HOURS:___

☐ GOOD DREAMS ☐ BAD DREAMS ☐ NO DREAMS

NOTES:

WHAT I ATE FOR:

BREAKFAST:	LUNCH:
DINNER:	SNACKS:

NUMBER OF CUPS OF WATER I DRANK:___

EXERCISE: ___:___ TO ___:___ MINUTES:___

TYPE:

OTHER ACTIVITIES:

☐ JOURNALING
☐ SOCIAL TIME
☐ MEDITATION
☐ GRATITUDE
☐ TIME OUTSIDE
☐ CREATIVE WORK
☐ SPIRITUAL PRACTICE
☐ SPA DAY
☐ THERAPY
☐ ALONE TIME
☐ BEING SILLY
☐ LEARNING SOMETHING NEW
☐ LISTENING TO MUSIC
☐ COOKING
☐ CLEANING
☐ ___________

REFLECT

PHYSICALLY, I FEEL:

- [ ] ENERGIZED
- [ ] WELL-RESTED
- [ ] STRONG
- [ ] LIMBER
- [ ] RELAXED
- [ ] ____________
- [ ] SLUGGISH
- [ ] TIRED
- [ ] WEAK
- [ ] SORE
- [ ] STRESSED
- [ ] ____________

THINGS THAT WERE FUN OR RELAXING TODAY:

____

____

____

THINGS THAT WERE HARD OR STRESSFUL TODAY:

____

____

____

OTHER THOUGHTS:

____

____

____

____

____

____

____

____

KIND THINGS I DID FOR MYSELF:

____

____

____

TIME:	AS I WOKE UP			AS I WENT TO SLEEP
MOOD:				
NOTES:				

RECORD

DATE ___/___/___

AN INTENTION FOR THE DAY:

SLEPT: FROM ___:___ TO ___:___ TOTAL HOURS:___

☐ GOOD DREAMS ☐ BAD DREAMS ☐ NO DREAMS

NOTES:

WHAT I ATE FOR:

BREAKFAST:	LUNCH:
DINNER:	SNACKS:

NUMBER OF CUPS OF WATER I DRANK: ___

EXERCISE: ___:___ TO ___:___ MINUTES:___

TYPE:

OTHER ACTIVITIES:

☐ JOURNALING
☐ SOCIAL TIME
☐ MEDITATION
☐ GRATITUDE
☐ TIME OUTSIDE
☐ CREATIVE WORK
☐ SPIRITUAL PRACTICE
☐ SPA DAY
☐ THERAPY
☐ ALONE TIME
☐ BEING SILLY
☐ LEARNING SOMETHING NEW
☐ LISTENING TO MUSIC
☐ COOKING
☐ CLEANING
☐ ___________

REFLECT

PHYSICALLY, I FEEL:

- [ ] ENERGIZED
- [ ] WELL-RESTED
- [ ] STRONG
- [ ] LIMBER
- [ ] RELAXED
- [ ] ____________
- [ ] SLUGGISH
- [ ] TIRED
- [ ] WEAK
- [ ] SORE
- [ ] STRESSED
- [ ] ____________

THINGS THAT WERE FUN OR RELAXING TODAY:

____

____

____

THINGS THAT WERE HARD OR STRESSFUL TODAY:

____

____

____

OTHER THOUGHTS:

____

____

____

____

____

____

____

____

KIND THINGS I DID FOR MYSELF:

____

____

____

TIME:	AS I WOKE UP			AS I WENT TO SLEEP
MOOD:				
NOTES:				

RECORD

DATE ___/___/___

AN INTENTION FOR THE DAY:

SLEPT: FROM ___:___ TO ___:___ TOTAL HOURS:___

☐ GOOD DREAMS ☐ BAD DREAMS ☐ NO DREAMS

NOTES:

WHAT I ATE FOR:

BREAKFAST:	LUNCH:
DINNER:	SNACKS:

NUMBER OF CUPS OF WATER I DRANK: ___

EXERCISE: ___:___ TO ___:___ MINUTES:___

TYPE:

OTHER ACTIVITIES:

☐ JOURNALING
☐ SOCIAL TIME
☐ MEDITATION
☐ GRATITUDE
☐ TIME OUTSIDE
☐ CREATIVE WORK
☐ SPIRITUAL PRACTICE
☐ SPA DAY
☐ THERAPY
☐ ALONE TIME
☐ BEING SILLY
☐ LEARNING SOMETHING NEW
☐ LISTENING TO MUSIC
☐ COOKING
☐ CLEANING
☐ ___________

REFLECT

PHYSICALLY, I FEEL:

- [ ] ENERGIZED
- [ ] WELL-RESTED
- [ ] STRONG
- [ ] LIMBER
- [ ] RELAXED
- [ ] ______________
- [ ] SLUGGISH
- [ ] TIRED
- [ ] WEAK
- [ ] SORE
- [ ] STRESSED
- [ ] ______________

THINGS THAT WERE FUN OR RELAXING TODAY:

____

____

____

THINGS THAT WERE HARD OR STRESSFUL TODAY:

____

____

____

OTHER THOUGHTS:

____

____

____

____

____

____

____

____

KIND THINGS I DID FOR MYSELF:

____

____

____

TIME:	AS I WOKE UP			AS I WENT TO SLEEP
MOOD:				
NOTES:				

RECORD

DATE ___/___/___

AN INTENTION FOR THE DAY:

SLEPT: FROM ___:___ TO ___:___ TOTAL HOURS:___

☐ GOOD DREAMS ☐ BAD DREAMS ☐ NO DREAMS

NOTES:

WHAT I ATE FOR:

BREAKFAST:	LUNCH:
DINNER:	SNACKS:

NUMBER OF CUPS OF WATER I DRANK:___

EXERCISE: ___:___ TO ___:___ MINUTES:___

TYPE:

OTHER ACTIVITIES:

☐ JOURNALING
☐ SOCIAL TIME
☐ MEDITATION
☐ GRATITUDE
☐ TIME OUTSIDE
☐ CREATIVE WORK
☐ SPIRITUAL PRACTICE
☐ SPA DAY
☐ THERAPY
☐ ALONE TIME
☐ BEING SILLY
☐ LEARNING SOMETHING NEW
☐ LISTENING TO MUSIC
☐ COOKING
☐ CLEANING
☐ ___________

REFLECT

PHYSICALLY, I FEEL:

- [ ] ENERGIZED
- [ ] WELL-RESTED
- [ ] STRONG
- [ ] LIMBER
- [ ] RELAXED
- [ ] ______________
- [ ] SLUGGISH
- [ ] TIRED
- [ ] WEAK
- [ ] SORE
- [ ] STRESSED
- [ ] ______________

THINGS THAT WERE FUN OR RELAXING TODAY:

____

____

____

THINGS THAT WERE HARD OR STRESSFUL TODAY:

____

____

____

OTHER THOUGHTS:

____

____

____

____

____

____

____

____

KIND THINGS I DID FOR MYSELF:

____

____

____

TIME:	AS I WOKE UP			AS I WENT TO SLEEP
MOOD:				
NOTES:				

RECORD

DATE ___/___/___

AN INTENTION FOR THE DAY:

SLEPT: FROM ___:___ TO ___:___ TOTAL HOURS:___

☐ GOOD DREAMS ☐ BAD DREAMS ☐ NO DREAMS

NOTES:

WHAT I ATE FOR:

BREAKFAST:	LUNCH:
DINNER:	SNACKS:

NUMBER OF CUPS OF WATER I DRANK:___

EXERCISE: ___:___ TO ___:___ MINUTES:___

TYPE:

OTHER ACTIVITIES:

- ☐ JOURNALING
- ☐ SOCIAL TIME
- ☐ MEDITATION
- ☐ GRATITUDE
- ☐ TIME OUTSIDE
- ☐ CREATIVE WORK
- ☐ SPIRITUAL PRACTICE
- ☐ SPA DAY
- ☐ THERAPY
- ☐ ALONE TIME
- ☐ BEING SILLY
- ☐ LEARNING SOMETHING NEW
- ☐ LISTENING TO MUSIC
- ☐ COOKING
- ☐ CLEANING
- ☐ ___________

REFLECT

PHYSICALLY, I FEEL:

☐ ENERGIZED	☐ SLUGGISH
☐ WELL-RESTED	☐ TIRED
☐ STRONG	☐ WEAK
☐ LIMBER	☐ SORE
☐ RELAXED	☐ STRESSED
☐ ______________	☐ ______________

THINGS THAT WERE FUN OR RELAXING TODAY:

____

____

____

THINGS THAT WERE HARD OR STRESSFUL TODAY:

____

____

____

OTHER THOUGHTS:

____

____

____

____

____

____

____

____

KIND THINGS I DID FOR MYSELF:

____

____

____

TIME:	AS I WOKE UP			AS I WENT TO SLEEP
MOOD:				
NOTES:				

RECORD

DATE ___/___/___

AN INTENTION FOR THE DAY:

SLEPT: FROM ___:___ TO ___:___ TOTAL HOURS:___

☐ GOOD DREAMS ☐ BAD DREAMS ☐ NO DREAMS

NOTES:

WHAT I ATE FOR:

BREAKFAST:	LUNCH:
DINNER:	SNACKS:

NUMBER OF CUPS OF WATER I DRANK:___

EXERCISE: ___:___ TO ___:___ MINUTES:___

TYPE:

OTHER ACTIVITIES:

- ☐ JOURNALING
- ☐ SOCIAL TIME
- ☐ MEDITATION
- ☐ GRATITUDE
- ☐ TIME OUTSIDE
- ☐ CREATIVE WORK
- ☐ SPIRITUAL PRACTICE
- ☐ SPA DAY
- ☐ THERAPY
- ☐ ALONE TIME
- ☐ BEING SILLY
- ☐ LEARNING SOMETHING NEW
- ☐ LISTENING TO MUSIC
- ☐ COOKING
- ☐ CLEANING
- ☐ ___________

REFLECT

PHYSICALLY, I FEEL:

☐ ENERGIZED
☐ WELL-RESTED
☐ STRONG
☐ LIMBER
☐ RELAXED
☐ ____________

☐ SLUGGISH
☐ TIRED
☐ WEAK
☐ SORE
☐ STRESSED
☐ ____________

THINGS THAT WERE FUN OR RELAXING TODAY:

____
____
____

THINGS THAT WERE HARD OR STRESSFUL TODAY:

____
____
____

OTHER THOUGHTS:

____
____
____
____
____
____
____
____

KIND THINGS I DID FOR MYSELF:

____
____
____

TIME:	AS I WOKE UP			AS I WENT TO SLEEP
MOOD:				
NOTES:				

RECORD

DATE ___/___/___

AN INTENTION FOR THE DAY:

SLEPT: FROM ___:___ TO ___:___ TOTAL HOURS:___

☐ GOOD DREAMS ☐ BAD DREAMS ☐ NO DREAMS

NOTES:

WHAT I ATE FOR:

BREAKFAST:	LUNCH:
DINNER:	SNACKS:

NUMBER OF CUPS OF WATER I DRANK:___

EXERCISE: ___:___ TO ___:___ MINUTES:___

TYPE:

OTHER ACTIVITIES:

☐ JOURNALING
☐ SOCIAL TIME
☐ MEDITATION
☐ GRATITUDE
☐ TIME OUTSIDE
☐ CREATIVE WORK
☐ SPIRITUAL PRACTICE
☐ SPA DAY
☐ THERAPY
☐ ALONE TIME
☐ BEING SILLY
☐ LEARNING SOMETHING NEW
☐ LISTENING TO MUSIC
☐ COOKING
☐ CLEANING
☐ ___

REFLECT

PHYSICALLY, I FEEL:

- [ ] ENERGIZED
- [ ] WELL-RESTED
- [ ] STRONG
- [ ] LIMBER
- [ ] RELAXED
- [ ] ______________
- [ ] SLUGGISH
- [ ] TIRED
- [ ] WEAK
- [ ] SORE
- [ ] STRESSED
- [ ] ______________

THINGS THAT WERE FUN OR RELAXING TODAY:

____

____

____

THINGS THAT WERE HARD OR STRESSFUL TODAY:

____

____

____

OTHER THOUGHTS:

____

____

____

____

____

____

____

____

KIND THINGS I DID FOR MYSELF:

____

____

____

TIME:	AS I WOKE UP			AS I WENT TO SLEEP
MOOD:				
NOTES:				

RECORD

DATE ___/___/___

AN INTENTION FOR THE DAY:

SLEPT: FROM ___:___ TO ___:___ TOTAL HOURS:___

☐ GOOD DREAMS ☐ BAD DREAMS ☐ NO DREAMS

NOTES:

WHAT I ATE FOR:

BREAKFAST:	LUNCH:
DINNER:	SNACKS:

NUMBER OF CUPS OF WATER I DRANK: ___

EXERCISE: ___:___ TO ___:___ MINUTES:___

TYPE:

OTHER ACTIVITIES:

☐ JOURNALING
☐ SOCIAL TIME
☐ MEDITATION
☐ GRATITUDE
☐ TIME OUTSIDE
☐ CREATIVE WORK
☐ SPIRITUAL PRACTICE
☐ SPA DAY
☐ THERAPY
☐ ALONE TIME
☐ BEING SILLY
☐ LEARNING SOMETHING NEW
☐ LISTENING TO MUSIC
☐ COOKING
☐ CLEANING
☐ ___________

REFLECT

PHYSICALLY, I FEEL:

- [ ] ENERGIZED
- [ ] WELL-RESTED
- [ ] STRONG
- [ ] LIMBER
- [ ] RELAXED
- [ ] ______________
- [ ] SLUGGISH
- [ ] TIRED
- [ ] WEAK
- [ ] SORE
- [ ] STRESSED
- [ ] ______________

THINGS THAT WERE FUN OR RELAXING TODAY:

____

____

____

THINGS THAT WERE HARD OR STRESSFUL TODAY:

____

____

____

OTHER THOUGHTS:

____

____

____

____

____

____

____

____

KIND THINGS I DID FOR MYSELF:

____

____

____

TIME:	AS I WOKE UP			AS I WENT TO SLEEP
MOOD:				
NOTES:				

RECORD

DATE ___/___/___

AN INTENTION FOR THE DAY:

SLEPT: FROM ___:___ TO ___:___ TOTAL HOURS: ___

☐ GOOD DREAMS ☐ BAD DREAMS ☐ NO DREAMS

NOTES:

WHAT I ATE FOR:

BREAKFAST:	LUNCH:
DINNER:	SNACKS:

NUMBER OF CUPS OF WATER I DRANK: ___

EXERCISE: ___:___ TO ___:___ MINUTES: ___

TYPE:

OTHER ACTIVITIES:

- ☐ JOURNALING
- ☐ SOCIAL TIME
- ☐ MEDITATION
- ☐ GRATITUDE
- ☐ TIME OUTSIDE
- ☐ CREATIVE WORK
- ☐ SPIRITUAL PRACTICE
- ☐ SPA DAY
- ☐ THERAPY
- ☐ ALONE TIME
- ☐ BEING SILLY
- ☐ LEARNING SOMETHING NEW
- ☐ LISTENING TO MUSIC
- ☐ COOKING
- ☐ CLEANING
- ☐ ___________

REFLECT

PHYSICALLY, I FEEL:

- [ ] ENERGIZED
- [ ] WELL-RESTED
- [ ] STRONG
- [ ] LIMBER
- [ ] RELAXED
- [ ] ____________
- [ ] SLUGGISH
- [ ] TIRED
- [ ] WEAK
- [ ] SORE
- [ ] STRESSED
- [ ] ____________

THINGS THAT WERE FUN OR RELAXING TODAY:

____

____

____

THINGS THAT WERE HARD OR STRESSFUL TODAY:

____

____

____

OTHER THOUGHTS:

____

____

____

____

____

____

____

____

KIND THINGS I DID FOR MYSELF:

____

____

____

TIME:	AS I WOKE UP			AS I WENT TO SLEEP
MOOD:				
NOTES:				

RECORD

DATE ___/___/___

AN INTENTION FOR THE DAY:

SLEPT: FROM ___:___ TO ___:___ TOTAL HOURS:___

☐ GOOD DREAMS ☐ BAD DREAMS ☐ NO DREAMS

NOTES:

WHAT I ATE FOR:

BREAKFAST:	LUNCH:
DINNER:	SNACKS:

NUMBER OF CUPS OF WATER I DRANK:___

EXERCISE: ___:___ TO ___:___ TOTAL MINUTES:___

TYPE:

OTHER ACTIVITIES:

☐ JOURNALING
☐ SOCIAL TIME
☐ MEDITATION
☐ GRATITUDE
☐ TIME OUTSIDE
☐ CREATIVE WORK
☐ SPIRITUAL PRACTICE
☐ SPA DAY
☐ THERAPY
☐ ALONE TIME
☐ BEING SILLY
☐ LEARNING SOMETHING NEW
☐ LISTENING TO MUSIC
☐ COOKING
☐ CLEANING
☐ ___

REFLECT

PHYSICALLY, I FEEL:

- [ ] ENERGIZED
- [ ] WELL-RESTED
- [ ] STRONG
- [ ] LIMBER
- [ ] RELAXED
- [ ] ______________
- [ ] SLUGGISH
- [ ] TIRED
- [ ] WEAK
- [ ] SORE
- [ ] STRESSED
- [ ] ______________

THINGS THAT WERE FUN OR RELAXING TODAY:

____

____

____

THINGS THAT WERE HARD OR STRESSFUL TODAY:

____

____

____

KIND THINGS I DID FOR MYSELF:

____

____

____

OTHER THOUGHTS:

TIME:	AS I WOKE UP			AS I WENT TO SLEEP
MOOD:				
NOTES:				

RECORD

DATE ___/___/___

AN INTENTION FOR THE DAY:

SLEPT: FROM ___:___ TO ___:___ TOTAL HOURS:___

☐ GOOD DREAMS ☐ BAD DREAMS ☐ NO DREAMS

NOTES:

WHAT I ATE FOR:

BREAKFAST:	LUNCH:
DINNER:	SNACKS:

NUMBER OF CUPS OF WATER I DRANK:___

EXERCISE: ___:___ TO ___:___ TOTAL MINUTES:___

TYPE:

OTHER ACTIVITIES:

☐ JOURNALING
☐ SOCIAL TIME
☐ MEDITATION
☐ GRATITUDE
☐ TIME OUTSIDE
☐ CREATIVE WORK
☐ SPIRITUAL PRACTICE
☐ SPA DAY
☐ THERAPY
☐ ALONE TIME
☐ BEING SILLY
☐ LEARNING SOMETHING NEW
☐ LISTENING TO MUSIC
☐ COOKING
☐ CLEANING
☐ ________

REFLECT

PHYSICALLY, I FEEL:

- ☐ ENERGIZED
- ☐ WELL-RESTED
- ☐ STRONG
- ☐ LIMBER
- ☐ RELAXED
- ☐ ____________
- ☐ SLUGGISH
- ☐ TIRED
- ☐ WEAK
- ☐ SORE
- ☐ STRESSED
- ☐ ____________

THINGS THAT WERE FUN OR RELAXING TODAY:

____

____

____

OTHER THOUGHTS:

THINGS THAT WERE HARD OR STRESSFUL TODAY:

____

____

____

KIND THINGS I DID FOR MYSELF:

____

____

____

TIME:	AS I WOKE UP			AS I WENT TO SLEEP
MOOD:				
NOTES:				

RECORD

DATE ___/___/___

AN INTENTION FOR THE DAY:

SLEPT: FROM ___:___ TO ___:___ TOTAL HOURS:___

☐ GOOD DREAMS ☐ BAD DREAMS ☐ NO DREAMS

NOTES:

WHAT I ATE FOR:

BREAKFAST:	LUNCH:
DINNER:	SNACKS:

NUMBER OF CUPS OF WATER I DRANK:___

EXERCISE: ___:___ TO ___:___ TOTAL MINUTES:___

TYPE:

OTHER ACTIVITIES:

☐ JOURNALING
☐ SOCIAL TIME
☐ MEDITATION
☐ GRATITUDE
☐ TIME OUTSIDE
☐ CREATIVE WORK
☐ SPIRITUAL PRACTICE
☐ SPA DAY
☐ THERAPY
☐ ALONE TIME
☐ BEING SILLY
☐ LEARNING SOMETHING NEW
☐ LISTENING TO MUSIC
☐ COOKING
☐ CLEANING
☐ ___________

REFLECT

PHYSICALLY, I FEEL:

- ☐ ENERGIZED
- ☐ WELL-RESTED
- ☐ STRONG
- ☐ LIMBER
- ☐ RELAXED
- ☐ ____________
- ☐ SLUGGISH
- ☐ TIRED
- ☐ WEAK
- ☐ SORE
- ☐ STRESSED
- ☐ ____________

THINGS THAT WERE FUN OR RELAXING TODAY:

____

____

____

OTHER THOUGHTS:

THINGS THAT WERE HARD OR STRESSFUL TODAY:

____

____

____

KIND THINGS I DID FOR MYSELF:

____

____

____

TIME:	AS I WOKE UP			AS I WENT TO SLEEP
MOOD:				
NOTES:				

RECORD

DATE ___/___/___

AN INTENTION FOR THE DAY:

SLEPT: FROM ___:___ TO ___:___ TOTAL HOURS:___

☐ GOOD DREAMS ☐ BAD DREAMS ☐ NO DREAMS

NOTES:

WHAT I ATE FOR:

BREAKFAST:	LUNCH:
DINNER:	SNACKS:

NUMBER OF CUPS OF WATER I DRANK:___

EXERCISE: ___:___ TO ___:___ TOTAL MINUTES:___

TYPE:

OTHER ACTIVITIES:

- ☐ JOURNALING
- ☐ SOCIAL TIME
- ☐ MEDITATION
- ☐ GRATITUDE
- ☐ TIME OUTSIDE
- ☐ CREATIVE WORK
- ☐ SPIRITUAL PRACTICE
- ☐ SPA DAY
- ☐ THERAPY
- ☐ ALONE TIME
- ☐ BEING SILLY
- ☐ LEARNING SOMETHING NEW
- ☐ LISTENING TO MUSIC
- ☐ COOKING
- ☐ CLEANING
- ☐ ___________

REFLECT

PHYSICALLY, I FEEL:

☐ ENERGIZED	☐ SLUGGISH
☐ WELL-RESTED	☐ TIRED
☐ STRONG	☐ WEAK
☐ LIMBER	☐ SORE
☐ RELAXED	☐ STRESSED
☐ ____________	☐ ____________

THINGS THAT WERE FUN OR RELAXING TODAY:

OTHER THOUGHTS:

THINGS THAT WERE HARD OR STRESSFUL TODAY:

KIND THINGS I DID FOR MYSELF:

TIME:	AS I WOKE UP			AS I WENT TO SLEEP
MOOD:				
NOTES:				

RECORD

DATE ___/___/___

AN INTENTION FOR THE DAY:

SLEPT: FROM ___:___ TO ___:___ TOTAL HOURS:___

☐ GOOD DREAMS ☐ BAD DREAMS ☐ NO DREAMS

NOTES:

WHAT I ATE FOR:

BREAKFAST:	LUNCH:
DINNER:	SNACKS:

NUMBER OF CUPS OF WATER I DRANK:___

EXERCISE: ___:___ TO ___:___ TOTAL MINUTES:___

TYPE:

OTHER ACTIVITIES:

☐ JOURNALING
☐ SOCIAL TIME
☐ MEDITATION
☐ GRATITUDE
☐ TIME OUTSIDE
☐ CREATIVE WORK
☐ SPIRITUAL PRACTICE
☐ SPA DAY
☐ THERAPY
☐ ALONE TIME
☐ BEING SILLY
☐ LEARNING SOMETHING NEW
☐ LISTENING TO MUSIC
☐ COOKING
☐ CLEANING
☐ ___________

REFLECT

PHYSICALLY, I FEEL:

- [ ] ENERGIZED
- [ ] WELL-RESTED
- [ ] STRONG
- [ ] LIMBER
- [ ] RELAXED
- [ ] ____________
- [ ] SLUGGISH
- [ ] TIRED
- [ ] WEAK
- [ ] SORE
- [ ] STRESSED
- [ ] ____________

THINGS THAT WERE FUN OR RELAXING TODAY:

____

____

____

OTHER THOUGHTS:

THINGS THAT WERE HARD OR STRESSFUL TODAY:

____

____

____

KIND THINGS I DID FOR MYSELF:

____

____

____

TIME:	AS I WOKE UP			AS I WENT TO SLEEP
MOOD:				
NOTES:				

RECORD

DATE ___/___/___

AN INTENTION FOR THE DAY:

SLEPT: FROM ___:___ TO ___:___ TOTAL HOURS: ___

☐ GOOD DREAMS ☐ BAD DREAMS ☐ NO DREAMS

NOTES:

WHAT I ATE FOR:

BREAKFAST:	LUNCH:
DINNER:	SNACKS:

NUMBER OF CUPS OF WATER I DRANK: ___

EXERCISE: ___:___ TO ___:___ TOTAL MINUTES: ___

TYPE:

OTHER ACTIVITIES:

- ☐ JOURNALING
- ☐ SOCIAL TIME
- ☐ MEDITATION
- ☐ GRATITUDE
- ☐ TIME OUTSIDE
- ☐ CREATIVE WORK
- ☐ SPIRITUAL PRACTICE
- ☐ SPA DAY
- ☐ THERAPY
- ☐ ALONE TIME
- ☐ BEING SILLY
- ☐ LEARNING SOMETHING NEW
- ☐ LISTENING TO MUSIC
- ☐ COOKING
- ☐ CLEANING
- ☐ ___________

REFLECT

PHYSICALLY, I FEEL:

- ☐ ENERGIZED
- ☐ WELL-RESTED
- ☐ STRONG
- ☐ LIMBER
- ☐ RELAXED
- ☐ ____________
- ☐ SLUGGISH
- ☐ TIRED
- ☐ WEAK
- ☐ SORE
- ☐ STRESSED
- ☐ ____________

THINGS THAT WERE FUN OR RELAXING TODAY:

____

____

____

THINGS THAT WERE HARD OR STRESSFUL TODAY:

____

____

____

KIND THINGS I DID FOR MYSELF:

____

____

____

OTHER THOUGHTS:

TIME:	AS I WOKE UP			AS I WENT TO SLEEP
MOOD:				
NOTES:				

RECORD

DATE ___/___/___

AN INTENTION FOR THE DAY:

SLEPT: FROM ___:___ TO ___:___ TOTAL HOURS:___

☐ GOOD DREAMS ☐ BAD DREAMS ☐ NO DREAMS

NOTES:

WHAT I ATE FOR:

BREAKFAST:	LUNCH:
DINNER:	SNACKS:

NUMBER OF CUPS OF WATER I DRANK:___

EXERCISE: ___:___ TO ___:___ TOTAL MINUTES:___

TYPE:

OTHER ACTIVITIES:

☐ JOURNALING
☐ SOCIAL TIME
☐ MEDITATION
☐ GRATITUDE
☐ TIME OUTSIDE
☐ CREATIVE WORK
☐ SPIRITUAL PRACTICE
☐ SPA DAY
☐ THERAPY
☐ ALONE TIME
☐ BEING SILLY
☐ LEARNING SOMETHING NEW
☐ LISTENING TO MUSIC
☐ COOKING
☐ CLEANING
☐ ___________

REFLECT

PHYSICALLY, I FEEL:

- [ ] ENERGIZED
- [ ] WELL-RESTED
- [ ] STRONG
- [ ] LIMBER
- [ ] RELAXED
- [ ] ____________
- [ ] SLUGGISH
- [ ] TIRED
- [ ] WEAK
- [ ] SORE
- [ ] STRESSED
- [ ] ____________

THINGS THAT WERE FUN OR RELAXING TODAY:

____

____

____

THINGS THAT WERE HARD OR STRESSFUL TODAY:

____

____

____

OTHER THOUGHTS:

KIND THINGS I DID FOR MYSELF:

____

____

____

TIME:	AS I WOKE UP			AS I WENT TO SLEEP
MOOD:				
NOTES:				

RECORD

DATE ___/___/___

AN INTENTION FOR THE DAY:

SLEPT: FROM ___:___ TO ___:___ TOTAL HOURS:___

☐ GOOD DREAMS ☐ BAD DREAMS ☐ NO DREAMS

NOTES:

WHAT I ATE FOR:

BREAKFAST:	LUNCH:
DINNER:	SNACKS:

NUMBER OF CUPS OF WATER I DRANK:___

EXERCISE: ___:___ TO ___:___ TOTAL MINUTES:___

TYPE:

OTHER ACTIVITIES:

- ☐ JOURNALING
- ☐ SOCIAL TIME
- ☐ MEDITATION
- ☐ GRATITUDE
- ☐ TIME OUTSIDE
- ☐ CREATIVE WORK
- ☐ SPIRITUAL PRACTICE
- ☐ SPA DAY
- ☐ THERAPY
- ☐ ALONE TIME
- ☐ BEING SILLY
- ☐ LEARNING SOMETHING NEW
- ☐ LISTENING TO MUSIC
- ☐ COOKING
- ☐ CLEANING
- ☐ ___________

REFLECT

PHYSICALLY, I FEEL:

☐ ENERGIZED ☐ SLUGGISH
☐ WELL-RESTED ☐ TIRED
☐ STRONG ☐ WEAK
☐ LIMBER ☐ SORE
☐ RELAXED ☐ STRESSED
☐ ______________ ☐ ______________

THINGS THAT WERE FUN OR RELAXING TODAY:

____
____
____

THINGS THAT WERE HARD OR STRESSFUL TODAY:

____
____
____

OTHER THOUGHTS:

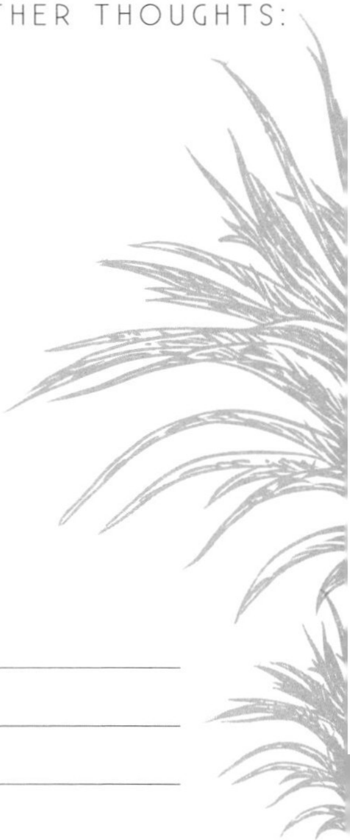

KIND THINGS I DID FOR MYSELF:

____
____
____

TIME:	AS I WOKE UP			AS I WENT TO SLEEP
MOOD:				
NOTES:				

RECORD

DATE ___/___/___

AN INTENTION FOR THE DAY:

SLEPT: FROM ___:___ TO ___:___ TOTAL HOURS:___

☐ GOOD DREAMS ☐ BAD DREAMS ☐ NO DREAMS

NOTES:

WHAT I ATE FOR:

BREAKFAST:	LUNCH:
DINNER:	SNACKS:

NUMBER OF CUPS OF WATER I DRANK:___

EXERCISE: ___:___ TO ___:___ TOTAL MINUTES:___

TYPE:

OTHER ACTIVITIES:

- ☐ JOURNALING
- ☐ SOCIAL TIME
- ☐ MEDITATION
- ☐ GRATITUDE
- ☐ TIME OUTSIDE
- ☐ CREATIVE WORK
- ☐ SPIRITUAL PRACTICE
- ☐ SPA DAY
- ☐ THERAPY
- ☐ ALONE TIME
- ☐ BEING SILLY
- ☐ LEARNING SOMETHING NEW
- ☐ LISTENING TO MUSIC
- ☐ COOKING
- ☐ CLEANING
- ☐ ___________

REFLECT

PHYSICALLY, I FEEL:

- ☐ ENERGIZED
- ☐ WELL-RESTED
- ☐ STRONG
- ☐ LIMBER
- ☐ RELAXED
- ☐ ________________
- ☐ SLUGGISH
- ☐ TIRED
- ☐ WEAK
- ☐ SORE
- ☐ STRESSED
- ☐ ________________

THINGS THAT WERE FUN OR RELAXING TODAY:

____

____

____

OTHER THOUGHTS:

THINGS THAT WERE HARD OR STRESSFUL TODAY:

____

____

____

KIND THINGS I DID FOR MYSELF:

____

____

____

TIME:	AS I WOKE UP			AS I WENT TO SLEEP
MOOD:				
NOTES:				

RECORD

DATE ___/___/___

AN INTENTION FOR THE DAY:

SLEPT: FROM ___:___ TO ___:___ TOTAL HOURS: ___

☐ GOOD DREAMS ☐ BAD DREAMS ☐ NO DREAMS

NOTES:

WHAT I ATE FOR:

BREAKFAST:	LUNCH:
DINNER:	SNACKS:

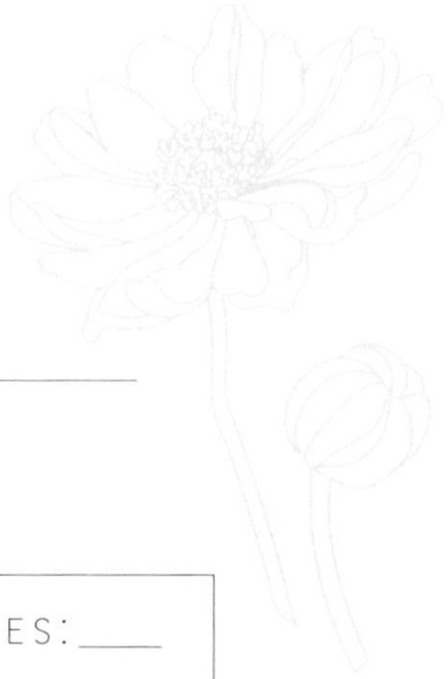

NUMBER OF CUPS OF WATER I DRANK: ___

EXERCISE: ___:___ TO ___:___ MINUTES: ___

TYPE:

OTHER ACTIVITIES:

- ☐ JOURNALING
- ☐ SOCIAL TIME
- ☐ MEDITATION
- ☐ GRATITUDE
- ☐ TIME OUTSIDE
- ☐ CREATIVE WORK
- ☐ SPIRITUAL PRACTICE
- ☐ SPA DAY
- ☐ THERAPY
- ☐ ALONE TIME
- ☐ BEING SILLY
- ☐ LEARNING SOMETHING NEW
- ☐ LISTENING TO MUSIC
- ☐ COOKING
- ☐ CLEANING
- ☐ ___________

REFLECT

PHYSICALLY, I FEEL:

- ☐ ENERGIZED
- ☐ WELL-RESTED
- ☐ STRONG
- ☐ LIMBER
- ☐ RELAXED
- ☐ ______
- ☐ SLUGGISH
- ☐ TIRED
- ☐ WEAK
- ☐ SORE
- ☐ STRESSED
- ☐ ______

THINGS THAT WERE FUN OR RELAXING TODAY:

THINGS THAT WERE HARD OR STRESSFUL TODAY:

OTHER THOUGHTS:

KIND THINGS I DID FOR MYSELF:

TIME:	AS I WOKE UP			AS I WENT TO SLEEP
MOOD:				
NOTES:				

RECORD

DATE ___/___/___

AN INTENTION FOR THE DAY:

SLEPT: FROM ___:___ TO ___:___ TOTAL HOURS:___

☐ GOOD DREAMS ☐ BAD DREAMS ☐ NO DREAMS

NOTES:

WHAT I ATE FOR:

BREAKFAST:	LUNCH:
DINNER:	SNACKS:

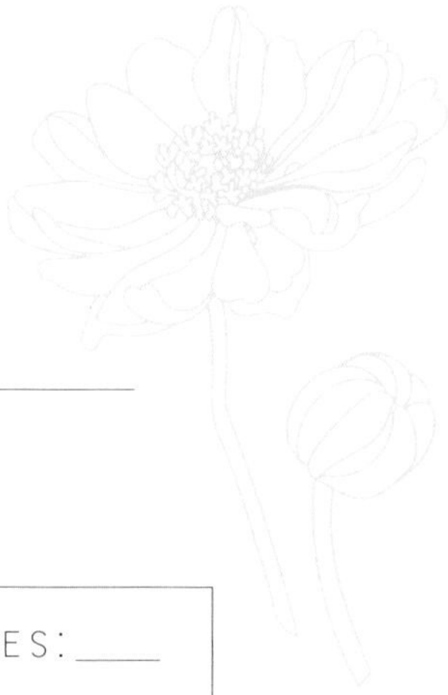

NUMBER OF CUPS OF WATER I DRANK:___

EXERCISE: ___:___ TO ___:___ MINUTES:___

TYPE:

OTHER ACTIVITIES:

- ☐ JOURNALING
- ☐ SOCIAL TIME
- ☐ MEDITATION
- ☐ GRATITUDE
- ☐ TIME OUTSIDE
- ☐ CREATIVE WORK
- ☐ SPIRITUAL PRACTICE
- ☐ SPA DAY
- ☐ THERAPY
- ☐ ALONE TIME
- ☐ BEING SILLY
- ☐ LEARNING SOMETHING NEW
- ☐ LISTENING TO MUSIC
- ☐ COOKING
- ☐ CLEANING
- ☐ ___________

REFLECT

PHYSICALLY, I FEEL:

- [ ] ENERGIZED
- [ ] WELL-RESTED
- [ ] STRONG
- [ ] LIMBER
- [ ] RELAXED
- [ ] ____________
- [ ] SLUGGISH
- [ ] TIRED
- [ ] WEAK
- [ ] SORE
- [ ] STRESSED
- [ ] ____________

THINGS THAT WERE FUN OR RELAXING TODAY:

OTHER THOUGHTS:

THINGS THAT WERE HARD OR STRESSFUL TODAY:

KIND THINGS I DID FOR MYSELF:

TIME:	AS I WOKE UP			AS I WENT TO SLEEP
MOOD:				
NOTES:				

RECORD

DATE ___/___/___

AN INTENTION FOR THE DAY:

SLEPT: FROM ___:___ TO ___:___ TOTAL HOURS:___

☐ GOOD DREAMS ☐ BAD DREAMS ☐ NO DREAMS

NOTES:

WHAT I ATE FOR:

BREAKFAST:	LUNCH:
DINNER:	SNACKS:

NUMBER OF CUPS OF WATER I DRANK:___

EXERCISE: ___:___ TO ___:___ MINUTES:___

TYPE:

OTHER ACTIVITIES:

- ☐ JOURNALING
- ☐ SOCIAL TIME
- ☐ MEDITATION
- ☐ GRATITUDE
- ☐ TIME OUTSIDE
- ☐ CREATIVE WORK
- ☐ SPIRITUAL PRACTICE
- ☐ SPA DAY
- ☐ THERAPY
- ☐ ALONE TIME
- ☐ BEING SILLY
- ☐ LEARNING SOMETHING NEW
- ☐ LISTENING TO MUSIC
- ☐ COOKING
- ☐ CLEANING
- ☐ ___________

REFLECT

PHYSICALLY, I FEEL:

- [ ] ENERGIZED
- [ ] WELL-RESTED
- [ ] STRONG
- [ ] LIMBER
- [ ] RELAXED
- [ ] ____________
- [ ] SLUGGISH
- [ ] TIRED
- [ ] WEAK
- [ ] SORE
- [ ] STRESSED
- [ ] ____________

THINGS THAT WERE FUN OR RELAXING TODAY:

THINGS THAT WERE HARD OR STRESSFUL TODAY:

OTHER THOUGHTS:

KIND THINGS I DID FOR MYSELF:

TIME:	AS I WOKE UP			AS I WENT TO SLEEP
MOOD:				
NOTES:				

RECORD

DATE ___/___/___

AN INTENTION FOR THE DAY:

SLEPT: FROM ___:___ TO ___:___ TOTAL HOURS: ___

☐ GOOD DREAMS ☐ BAD DREAMS ☐ NO DREAMS

NOTES:

WHAT I ATE FOR:

BREAKFAST:	LUNCH:
DINNER:	SNACKS:

NUMBER OF CUPS OF WATER I DRANK: ___

EXERCISE: ___:___ TO ___:___ MINUTES: ___

TYPE:

OTHER ACTIVITIES:

- ☐ JOURNALING
- ☐ SOCIAL TIME
- ☐ MEDITATION
- ☐ GRATITUDE
- ☐ TIME OUTSIDE
- ☐ CREATIVE WORK
- ☐ SPIRITUAL PRACTICE
- ☐ SPA DAY
- ☐ THERAPY
- ☐ ALONE TIME
- ☐ BEING SILLY
- ☐ LEARNING SOMETHING NEW
- ☐ LISTENING TO MUSIC
- ☐ COOKING
- ☐ CLEANING
- ☐ ___________

REFLECT

PHYSICALLY, I FEEL:

- [ ] ENERGIZED
- [ ] WELL-RESTED
- [ ] STRONG
- [ ] LIMBER
- [ ] RELAXED
- [ ] ______________
- [ ] SLUGGISH
- [ ] TIRED
- [ ] WEAK
- [ ] SORE
- [ ] STRESSED
- [ ] ______________

THINGS THAT WERE FUN OR RELAXING TODAY:

____

____

____

THINGS THAT WERE HARD OR STRESSFUL TODAY:

____

____

____

OTHER THOUGHTS:

KIND THINGS I DID FOR MYSELF:

____

____

____

TIME:	AS I WOKE UP			AS I WENT TO SLEEP
MOOD:				
NOTES:				

RECORD

DATE ___/___/___

AN INTENTION FOR THE DAY:

SLEPT: FROM ___:___ TO ___:___ TOTAL HOURS: ___

☐ GOOD DREAMS ☐ BAD DREAMS ☐ NO DREAMS

NOTES:

WHAT I ATE FOR:

BREAKFAST:	LUNCH:
DINNER:	SNACKS:

NUMBER OF CUPS OF WATER I DRANK: ___

EXERCISE: ___:___ TO ___:___ MINUTES: ___

TYPE:

OTHER ACTIVITIES:

- ☐ JOURNALING
- ☐ SOCIAL TIME
- ☐ MEDITATION
- ☐ GRATITUDE
- ☐ TIME OUTSIDE
- ☐ CREATIVE WORK
- ☐ SPIRITUAL PRACTICE
- ☐ SPA DAY
- ☐ THERAPY
- ☐ ALONE TIME
- ☐ BEING SILLY
- ☐ LEARNING SOMETHING NEW
- ☐ LISTENING TO MUSIC
- ☐ COOKING
- ☐ CLEANING
- ☐ ___

REFLECT

PHYSICALLY, I FEEL:

☐ ENERGIZED	☐ SLUGGISH
☐ WELL-RESTED	☐ TIRED
☐ STRONG	☐ WEAK
☐ LIMBER	☐ SORE
☐ RELAXED	☐ STRESSED
☐ ________________	☐ ________________

THINGS THAT WERE FUN OR RELAXING TODAY:

____

____

____

THINGS THAT WERE HARD OR STRESSFUL TODAY:

____

____

____

OTHER THOUGHTS:

KIND THINGS I DID FOR MYSELF:

____

____

____

TIME:	AS I WOKE UP			AS I WENT TO SLEEP
MOOD:				
NOTES:				

RECORD

DATE ___/___/___

AN INTENTION FOR THE DAY:

SLEPT: FROM ___:___ TO ___:___ TOTAL HOURS: ___

☐ GOOD DREAMS ☐ BAD DREAMS ☐ NO DREAMS

NOTES:

WHAT I ATE FOR:

BREAKFAST:	LUNCH:
DINNER:	SNACKS:

NUMBER OF CUPS OF WATER I DRANK: ___

EXERCISE: ___:___ TO ___:___ MINUTES: ___

TYPE:

OTHER ACTIVITIES:

- ☐ JOURNALING
- ☐ SOCIAL TIME
- ☐ MEDITATION
- ☐ GRATITUDE
- ☐ TIME OUTSIDE
- ☐ CREATIVE WORK
- ☐ SPIRITUAL PRACTICE
- ☐ SPA DAY
- ☐ THERAPY
- ☐ ALONE TIME
- ☐ BEING SILLY
- ☐ LEARNING SOMETHING NEW
- ☐ LISTENING TO MUSIC
- ☐ COOKING
- ☐ CLEANING
- ☐ ___________

REFLECT

PHYSICALLY, I FEEL:

☐ ENERGIZED	☐ SLUGGISH
☐ WELL-RESTED	☐ TIRED
☐ STRONG	☐ WEAK
☐ LIMBER	☐ SORE
☐ RELAXED	☐ STRESSED
☐ ____________	☐ ____________

THINGS THAT WERE FUN OR RELAXING TODAY:

THINGS THAT WERE HARD OR STRESSFUL TODAY:

OTHER THOUGHTS:

KIND THINGS I DID FOR MYSELF:

TIME:	AS I WOKE UP			AS I WENT TO SLEEP
MOOD:				
NOTES:				

RECORD

DATE ___/___/___

AN INTENTION FOR THE DAY:

SLEPT: FROM ___:___ TO ___:___ TOTAL HOURS: ___

☐ GOOD DREAMS ☐ BAD DREAMS ☐ NO DREAMS

NOTES:

WHAT I ATE FOR:

BREAKFAST:	LUNCH:
DINNER:	SNACKS:

NUMBER OF CUPS OF WATER I DRANK: ___

EXERCISE: ___:___ TO ___:___ MINUTES: ___

TYPE:

OTHER ACTIVITIES:

☐ JOURNALING

☐ SOCIAL TIME

☐ MEDITATION

☐ GRATITUDE

☐ TIME OUTSIDE

☐ CREATIVE WORK

☐ SPIRITUAL PRACTICE

☐ SPA DAY

☐ THERAPY

☐ ALONE TIME

☐ BEING SILLY

☐ LEARNING SOMETHING NEW

☐ LISTENING TO MUSIC

☐ COOKING

☐ CLEANING

☐ ______

REFLECT

PHYSICALLY, I FEEL:

- [ ] ENERGIZED
- [ ] WELL-RESTED
- [ ] STRONG
- [ ] LIMBER
- [ ] RELAXED
- [ ] ______________
- [ ] SLUGGISH
- [ ] TIRED
- [ ] WEAK
- [ ] SORE
- [ ] STRESSED
- [ ] ______________

THINGS THAT WERE FUN OR RELAXING TODAY:

____

____

____

THINGS THAT WERE HARD OR STRESSFUL TODAY:

____

____

____

OTHER THOUGHTS:

KIND THINGS I DID FOR MYSELF:

____

____

____

TIME:	AS I WOKE UP			AS I WENT TO SLEEP
MOOD:				
NOTES:				

RECORD

DATE ___/___/___

AN INTENTION FOR THE DAY:

SLEPT: FROM ___:___ TO ___:___ TOTAL HOURS: ___

☐ GOOD DREAMS ☐ BAD DREAMS ☐ NO DREAMS

NOTES:

WHAT I ATE FOR:

BREAKFAST:	LUNCH:
DINNER:	SNACKS:

NUMBER OF CUPS OF WATER I DRANK: ___

EXERCISE: ___:___ TO ___:___ MINUTES: ___

TYPE:

OTHER ACTIVITIES:

- ☐ JOURNALING
- ☐ SOCIAL TIME
- ☐ MEDITATION
- ☐ GRATITUDE
- ☐ TIME OUTSIDE
- ☐ CREATIVE WORK
- ☐ SPIRITUAL PRACTICE
- ☐ SPA DAY
- ☐ THERAPY
- ☐ ALONE TIME
- ☐ BEING SILLY
- ☐ LEARNING SOMETHING NEW
- ☐ LISTENING TO MUSIC
- ☐ COOKING
- ☐ CLEANING
- ☐ ___

REFLECT

PHYSICALLY, I FEEL:

- ☐ ENERGIZED
- ☐ WELL-RESTED
- ☐ STRONG
- ☐ LIMBER
- ☐ RELAXED
- ☐ ______________
- ☐ SLUGGISH
- ☐ TIRED
- ☐ WEAK
- ☐ SORE
- ☐ STRESSED
- ☐ ______________

THINGS THAT WERE FUN OR RELAXING TODAY:

____

____

____

THINGS THAT WERE HARD OR STRESSFUL TODAY:

____

____

____

OTHER THOUGHTS:

KIND THINGS I DID FOR MYSELF:

____

____

____

TIME:	AS I WOKE UP			AS I WENT TO SLEEP
MOOD:				
NOTES:				

RECORD

DATE ___/___/___

AN INTENTION FOR THE DAY:

SLEPT: FROM ____:____ TO ____:____ TOTAL HOURS:____

☐ GOOD DREAMS ☐ BAD DREAMS ☐ NO DREAMS

NOTES:

WHAT I ATE FOR:

BREAKFAST:	LUNCH:
DINNER:	SNACKS:

NUMBER OF CUPS OF WATER I DRANK:____

EXERCISE: ____:____ TO ____:____ MINUTES:____
TYPE:

OTHER ACTIVITIES:

☐ JOURNALING
☐ SOCIAL TIME
☐ MEDITATION
☐ GRATITUDE
☐ TIME OUTSIDE
☐ CREATIVE WORK
☐ SPIRITUAL PRACTICE
☐ SPA DAY
☐ THERAPY
☐ ALONE TIME
☐ BEING SILLY
☐ LEARNING SOMETHING NEW
☐ LISTENING TO MUSIC
☐ COOKING
☐ CLEANING
☐ ____________

REFLECT

PHYSICALLY, I FEEL:

- [ ] ENERGIZED
- [ ] WELL-RESTED
- [ ] STRONG
- [ ] LIMBER
- [ ] RELAXED
- [ ] ______________
- [ ] SLUGGISH
- [ ] TIRED
- [ ] WEAK
- [ ] SORE
- [ ] STRESSED
- [ ] ______________

THINGS THAT WERE FUN OR RELAXING TODAY:

____

____

____

THINGS THAT WERE HARD OR STRESSFUL TODAY:

____

____

____

OTHER THOUGHTS:

KIND THINGS I DID FOR MYSELF:

____

____

____

TIME:	AS I WOKE UP			AS I WENT TO SLEEP
MOOD:				
NOTES:				

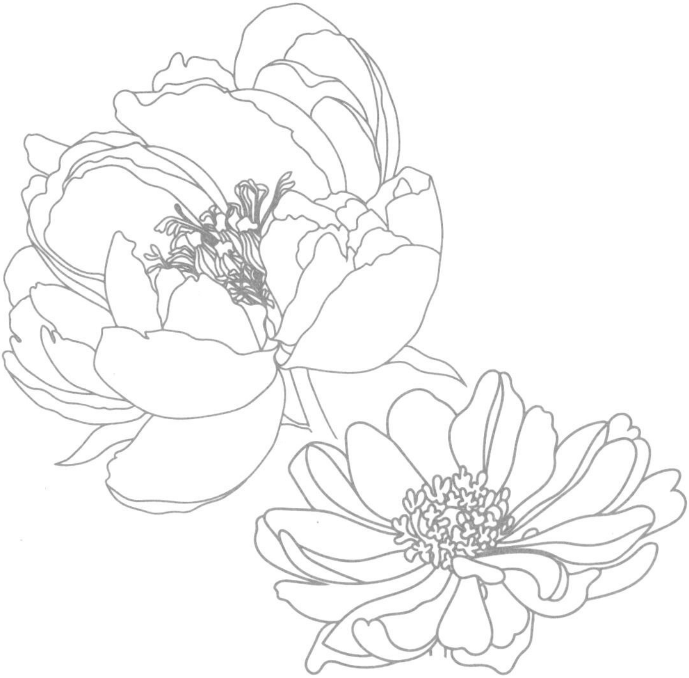

INSIGHTS

A Mandala Journal

MANDALA PUBLISHING

www.mandalaearth.com

MANUFACTURED IN CHINA

20 19 18 17 16 15 14